HEARTBREAK

HEARTBREAK

NEW APPROACHES TO HEALING

Recovering from lost love and mourning

GINETTE PARIS, PH.D.

WORLD BOOKS COLLECTIVE

Mill City Press
Minneapolis, MN

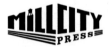

Mill City Press, Inc.

212 3rd Avenue North, Suite 290

Minneapolis, MN 55401

612.455.2294

www.millcitypublishing.com

ISBN-13: 978-1-936780-31-0

LCCN: 2011926463

Cover Design and Typeset by Sophie Chi

Printed in the United States of America

Praise for Ginette Paris:
Wisdom of the Psyche

"Emotionally personal, immediately useful, surprisingly original, beautifully deep, this page-turning read also turns the page into a new century of psychology. What an achievement."

> James Hillman, author *of Re-Visioning Psychology,* and of *The Soul's Code.*

ଔ

"Once again Ginette Paris demonstrates that she is quite simply the most original and eloquent of all writers on contemporary depth psychology."

> Michael Vannoy Adams, author of *The Mythological Unconscious*, and of *The Fantasy Principle.*

ଔ

"An extremely intelligent analysis and critique of the field of psychology today, both within and without academia. […] Full of brilliant, often poetic, nuggets of wisdom and insight that both startle and satisfy the reader eager for new or original ways to envision psychological reality."

> Jan Bauer, author of *Women and Alcoholism* and *Impossible Love.*

" The bright book of the future for everyone involved with depth psychology and its creative transformation of the arts and sciences. Ginette Paris's stunning achievement ... essential reading for the twenty-first century. We are all the richer for it."

Susan Rowland, author of Jung: a Feminist Revision, and
of C.G. Jung in the Humanities: Taking the Soul's Path

ଌ

"Every once in a rare while a book comes into one's hands that is so satisfying that it's hard to write about it without drenching every sentence in superlatives. This is such a book. [...] She speaks to us with controlled passion and dry, sparkling wit. [...]Paris is one of the most concise and articulate observer/critics of the culture in general and psychology in general, and one of the few who offers a corrective vision, and a wider one: we are encouraged to look to other disciplines to understand our own."

Lynn Cowan, author of Tracking the White Rabbit: A Subversive
View of Modern Culture and of Masochism: A Jungian View

ଌ

"[Paris's writing] stirs the depths of the soul even before it touches the surface of the mind. [...] She has de-schooled depth psychology and in her work of clearing away the jargon, she has bought the theories of depth psychology back home to the soul from which they have come. This is a rare achievement in psychological writing. Her book is an exercise in homecoming."

Robert D. Romanyshyn, author of The Soul in Grief:
Love, Death, and Transformation and of The Wounded
Researcher: Research with Soul in Mind.

"A fascinating book, with many layers of meaning. The elegance of her style [...] gives us a taste of the awe inspiring mysteries of life and how the present models of psychotherapy (medical, financial and redemptive) work against this ability to find a deeper meaning in life. [her writing] has the power to encourage one to participate in "amor fati", the love of one's fate, to endure the absurd, to cope with the insufferable, to lose one's innocence, and to embrace the totality of one's story as it unfolds. A brilliant look [...] enlarging our consciousness."

Maureen Murdock, author of the *Heroine's Journey*, and of *Father's Daughters.*

ACKNOWLEDGMENTS

I am forever grateful to those friends, colleagues and family members who gave helpful comments on various parts of this book: Linda Carter, Chris Clogston, Zenon-Gilles Maheu, Jan Marlan, Maureen Murdock, Lori Pye, Dennis Slattery.

I would also like to thank those friends, students, and patients who told me their stories, so that I could write the little vignettes all through this book. I cannot name them, but they will recognize our writing with four hands.

OTHER BOOKS BY GINETTE PARIS

- *The Wisdom of the Psyche: Depth Psychology after Neuroscience.* Routledge 2007.

- *The Psychology of Abortion.* Spring Publications 2007

- *Pagan Grace.* Spring Publications, 1990.

- *Pagan Meditations.* Spring Publications, 1986.

TABLE OF CONTENT

Where is the lover I knew? Ah! He has ridden off! Oh! Who will love me? AH! The woods are burgeoning all over, I am pining for my lover. The woods are turning green all over, why is my lover away so long? Ah! He has ridden off, Oh woe, who will love me? Ah!

Carmina Burana, a twelfth century song[1]

The lights in the harbor don't shine for me. I'm like a lost ship adrift on the sea. The sea of heartbreak. Lost love and loneliness. Memories of your caresses so divine, how I wish you were mine again my dear. I am on this sea of tears. Sea of heartbreak Oh, how did I lose you? Oh, where did I fail? Why did you leave me?

Lyrics of the song Sea of Heartbreak written in the twentieth century[2]

INTRODUCTION

Imagination and thought are admirable tools,
but they can be off. Suffering turns them on.

Marcel Proust[3]

Stated simply, the regulation of gene expression
by social factors makes all bodily functions,
including all functions of the brain, susceptible
to social influences. These social influences
will be biologically incorporated in the altered
expressions of specific genes in specific nerve
cells of specific regions of the brain. These
socially influenced alterations are transmitted
culturally. They are not incorporated in
the sperm and egg and therefore are not
transmitted genetically.

Kandel, E. 1998

There is a great deal of pain in life and perhaps the only pain
that can be avoided is the pain that comes from living with
a captive heart.

Nothing that happens to us, even the most terrible
shock, is unusable. A heartbreak is a master teacher: it can
show us not only the way to avoid the very serious medical

consequences of a loss of love, but it can also *force* us to recognize the deepest and darkest aspects of human love, a most valuable lesson if one wants to remain a person capable of loving. When something in us creates darkness, it sometimes radiates a somber serenity, like the night sky. That which brings darkness also offers the possibility of wisdom, if we do the work.

The psychic pain of mourning and heartbreak is truly unbearable, with all of the neurobiological evidence of a stress similar to being submitted to torture. There seems to be only one way to end that agony and limit the somatic damage: neuroscientists call it an *evolutionary jump,* while psychologists call it an *increase in consciousness.* What, one might ask, am I supposed to become conscious of? The answer is simple: you must look into the face of that irrational but very real fear that equates the partner's abandonment with death. It does not matter if what you fear is psychic death or physical death because the brain does not really differentiate between the two: psyche and soma are so intimately connected that psychic numbness *inevitably* leads to physical symptoms if you don't find the way back to joy. To become conscious of the irrational fear (the "don't leave me or I'll die" kind of feeling) poses a logical challenge, because to get rid of the fear you must learn to survive without the partner, which is precisely what you are terrified of! You are like a patient who has been shot by an arrow, but is afraid to let the doctor pull it out; living with an arrow sticking out from your chest makes life impossible.

What neuroscience calls an *evolutionary jump* defines the process that needs to happen for you now, to limit somatic damage. Whenever an intense effort of adaptation is required, following a radical and threatening change in our environment, either we "jump" to use the jargon of neuroscientists, or we regress and get sick. Just as early humans had to adapt to changes in climate and diet, today's humans constantly have to adapt to changes in the culture, crisis in the economy, storms in their psychological environment and, from time to time when the crisis is severe, a whole group will *jump* a rung on the ladder of evolution and invent something that will help them survive. Heartbreak qualifies as a major disruption to your psychic environment, and if you shut down instead of evolving, you'll suffer the repeated biochemical assaults that wear down the body/psyche connection. That is why the word *jump* combined with *evolutionary*, is just the right wording to define the healing process of heartbreak-through. Recovery is *not,* as so many are tempted to believe, a simple decision to "move on," which too often leads to an emotional shutting down, the closing of the heart. The *evolutionary jump*, paradoxically, happens only if the heart continues its painful expansion, and stays open until one learns something crucial about love and relationships.

There is a terrible waste in not harvesting the fruits of a devastating heartbreak. We know that the brain's fertility lies in its capacity to create new neuronal pathways, but the brain obliges only in response to situations that threaten; if your brain doesn't feel the threat, it won't bother to evolve.

Human evolution seems to follow common sense: if it works, don't fix it, but if there is a threat, get to work, fast and focused. Abandonment by, or death of the partner is one of the most intolerable threat to the human heart, and it is interpreted by the brain as a situation that asks for urgent re-alignment of neuronal activity. Your pain, if you can tolerate it without acting out in fear, will force you out of your dangerous psychic inferno.

Having survived the crossing of that desert, I wish to communicate my surprise and delight at the following discovery: when the heart is in prison, the mind can open a window! In my own situation of heartbreak I felt there was not much of a choice, as the torture was so intolerable that *something* had to happen. In my experience of grief, when my body could no longer endure the repeated biochemical assaults, I immersed myself in the study of the neuropsychology of heartbreak; I needed to understand what was the mess in my brain that made me cognitively impaired, depressed and panicky, with suicidal ideation and bouts of uncontrollable anger. This book, as well as the bibliography at the end, summarizes my intellectual and emotional trajectory through both the science and the psychology of grief. Neuroscience showed me *how* and *why* my painful loss was *forcing* me to evolve, while the depth psychological perspective offered me a *map* for figuring my way out. I did not have much of a choice: either I found something interesting and worthwhile in my story of heartbreak, or I remained stuck in the same sad lost-love song, like a CD on repeat mode. I feared the fate of someone living with a closed heart, a fate that would have robbed me of the wish to live.

I am writing from three different points of view:

1) First, as a teacher and researcher in psychology, I have spent most of my adult life studying the symptoms of lost love, tortuous love, smothering love, condemning love, controlling love, insufficient love, betrayed love, compulsive love, fusional/codependent love. I have studied and taught the theories that present themselves as antidotes to these poisons. This book is my summary and report from the field, at a time when scientific psychology is merging with neuroscience. I find it timely: neuroscience is debunking the pseudo-scientific claims of egomaniacal psychologists whose primary aim is to sell their copyrighted approach to the psyche. I mistrust those who sell recipes for conflict-free relationships and easy recovery, as if heartbreak were easy to fix with a few sanctimonious admonitions to "move on" and "stop being a co-dependent," promising recovery in ten easy lessons! Neuroscience invalidates those theories that have cheapened a true psychological approach, while it validates some crucial ideas from *depth psychology*, the branch of psychology that has historically allied itself with the humanities. *Depth psychology*, which means a psychology that takes into account the unconscious aspects of our brain, (what neuroscience calls *implicit memory*), comes in many flavors: Freudian and post-Freudian psychoanalysis, Jungian and post-Jungian, analytical psychology, archetypal

psychology, existential psychology, imaginal psychology, transpersonal psychology, eco-psychology… the brand name does not matter that much, for what I am interested in is how well psychological intuition will offer what science can never deliver: an initiation into the darker aspects of love and love-sickness.

2) Second, I am writing as a therapist, *listening* to the stories of courageous individuals free falling from the summit of love, crashing down into the relational desert of mourning, grief and loss. While witnessing their despair, I admired the courage it takes to survive heartbreak. Love, its presence and absence, quality and quantity, form and essence, its nurturing and toxic effects, its bitterness and sweetness, is at the core of *every* therapy, because love is fundamentally liberating. Yet love is also easily corrupted. Love develops the brain, but a heartbreak transforms an otherwise functional adult into a cognitive dimwit. Love attaches itself to our neurotic traits, which then develop like barnacles under the hull of a boat. For this book I interviewed patients, students, friends and colleagues to collect their stories of heartbreak and mourning. In collaboration with them, I wrote short vignettes, editing, pruning, condensing their narratives, offering a repertoire of metaphors ("is it *like* this, or *like* that…"), trying to reach a formulation that skips the details of their heartbreaks while communicating the archetypal essence of this torture. My project was to translate the inchoate moaning of their broken hearts into a minimal form of literature, finding the right

symbol, the right image for their misery. This was time spent *formulating,* which means finding the right *form*, the right fit between their emotional experiences and my limited literary capacities. Once we reached the point where the patient, friend, student, colleague, would say: "Yes, that's it, this is a good picture of my experience..." I pushed "command/ save" on the keyboard. Call it 'literary-therapy' if you will, the basic idea of those vignettes is to get at the depth of feelings, in order to reveal the archetypal core common to all heartbreaks, thus relieving some of the guilt associated to a failure of love.

3) And last, I am writing as a woman who has suffered her fair share of heartbreaks. As a young woman, I plunged into the cavernous mouth of that mythical beast we call Love, like a frog jumping into the path of a lawnmower. My heart was shredded, devoured, digested by the other, its substance giving him the energy to spit me out like the pit of a sweet date, and giving myself an excellent first lesson about the difference between the sweetness of love and the tragedy of remaining innocent about its power. As an *almost* old woman now, having lost some of my innocence and with a life-time of witnessing courageous individuals outwitting that same cruel beast, I am convinced that the person suffering the torture of heartbreak *can*, and *should*, be helped by all possible means: neuroscience and literature, medication and meditation, people and films, massages and humor, friendship and therapy, deep thinking and depth psychology. I have experienced the unbearable pain of

HEARTBREAK

heartbreak, and was not surprised to discover that it has all the neurobiological evidence of traumatic shock. Yet, my grief was also an extraordinary chance for an initiation into a deeper level of the reality of love.

The good news is this: if you love, your heart *should* and *will* be broken at some point or other in your life. If not, your love may remain the innocent love of a child.

Don't brag that you never experienced heartbreak; it may indicate that you have no heart to break!

CHAPTER 1

THE HEART AND THE BRAIN TEACH EACH OTHER

> *In the past century, there was an unfortunate division between the subject matter of neuropsychology and the lived reality of the mind. This once prompted the neurologist Oliver Sacks to write that "neuropsychology is admirable, but it excludes the psyche"! Happily that situation has now changed.*
>
> Mark Solms[4]

The first neurological reality I discovered is a simple one: life without the partner takes a huge effort of adaptation, like a right-handed person whose right hand is amputated, who now must learn to do everything with the left hand, with the whole brain having to re-configure its connections. The same is true when you are cut off from a partner; your brain *literally* has to reconfigure its connections. Until your brain is done with this updating, consider yourself handicapped: physically, emotionally, cognitively. Your brain needs time, and good conditions, to do its work, and you have to be patient and compassionate with yourself, just like you would be with somebody in rehab after a stroke. Chapter three and chapter four summarize the neuroscientific explanations for your temporary handicap; you may skip them if you already understand how neurogenesis occurs, or fails to occur.

The second reality from neuroscience that was truly helpful for me was the affirmation that the memory of a traumatic experience (like the loss of your partner) cannot be erased from the folds of your brain. In other words, it does not work to try to *forget* the relationship, its beauty, or its pain. One can only *add new aptitudes* to the repertoire of responses, and these new responses, over time, will over-ride the earlier ones.

The third neuroscientific reality I considered anew is one I already knew from my training as a psychologist: since love is the most profound bond between humans, it follows that its breakdown is the most devastating experience that the human heart can endure. This is true of *any* intimate connection, whether the relationship between lovers or that between parents and children. Parents have heartbreaks over their children just as children can be heartbroken by the indifference or abuse of a parent. Many shrivel and die because their first taste of love ended in rejection, loss, betrayal or abandonment, and, from then on, they denied themselves the primal waters of love. What kills them is not the betrayal or the loss, but the shutting down, the somatic deterioration, the addictions, and the psychic imprisonment in a dead or abusive relationship. My heartbreak was not over an abusive relationship, yet, I did feel the danger of never getting over it, and thus living in a loveless desert.

This book combines some of the major discoveries of neuroscience with the insights of psychology in order to convince you, the heartbroken person, to consider your pain as a necessary *push from nature*. In other words, your painful feelings contain the energy to propel you beyond your current state of devastation. Don't deny the pain, but sit instead in silence, feel it, suffer it, analyze it, become interested in it, and study the many psychological maps that lead out of this prison of the heart. No one volunteers for such an experience; yet, it happens, it is dangerous, and you need to take it seriously.

If the loss is due to the death of the Beloved, as opposed to separation or divorce, there is a kind of paradoxical advantage: you won't get stuck in failing schemes and strategies to regain the lost love. You know, right from the start, that there is no coming back on the part of he dead partner. Nevertheless, the danger of remaining stuck exists, but it takes the form of a fixation on the idealized dead partner, with whom, of course, no living person can ever compete, thus leaving the bereaved with the frustration of living with a ghost, stuck in the past, trying to entertain somebody who left. I have never met anyone who was helped by the stock advice to "just move on." This kind of advice feels to the heartbroken individual like an offending proposition. Nothing means anything anymore, so what good does it do to be told to *move on*? "Move... where?

Move... how? And why move at all? " The entire emotional landscape of the bereaved has been destroyed. Depression is a state of utter stagnation, an absence of movement; being told to *move on* is like telling a mourner to cheer up. Many theories about mourning consider recovery from the point of view of *stages*: a one-year cycle of mourning is supposed to heal the heart, a point of view adopted by the DSM IV. Technically speaking, if you are depressed for three hundred and sixty-five days after the death of your partner, a psychiatric evaluation can still consider you "normal"; but more than that (how about three hundred and sixty-six days?) it is supposed to indicate "pathological mourning" . Your grief, according to the DSM-IV, falls into the clinical category of "Adjustment Disorder." [1] I don't know any competent psychotherapist who shows that kind of rigidity in diagnosis, because individuals don't all mourn at the same speed. A suggestion has been made by the DSM researchers that a new category should be added to the next edition of the DSM: *Complicated Grief Disorder*. The proposed diagnostic criteria describe bereavement that lasts more than 14 months, "with a severity that interferes with daily functioning and with any three of the following seven symptoms: 1) Unbidden memories or intrusive fantasies related to the lost relationship. 2) Strong spells or pangs of severe emotion related to the lost relationship. 3) Distressingly strong yearnings or wishes that the deceased were there. 4) Feelings of being far too much alone or personally empty. 5) Excessively staying away from people,

places, or activities that remind the subject of the deceased
6) Unusual levels of sleep interference. 7) Loss of interest
in work, social, caretaking, or recreational activities to a
maladaptive degree." [2] In short, psychiatry is describing, in
clinical terms, the *absolute misery* that every lost-love song
has described since poetry and song came into existence; in
a nutshell, psychiatry is saying: the misery of grief can last
for a shorter or longer period, and if it goes on for too long,
life loses its appeal.

The broken hearted person needs something more than
a good diagnosis, which in turn can lead to medication,
which is what the DSM can offer. Medication can help
with the anxiety and insomnia, but it is not until you have
a completely new identity, a new story line that you will
get over the loss. One of the reasons we enjoy reading
novels and watching movies is that we are presented with
a plot in which the *outer action* (the *moves* in the *movie*)
has the capacity to resolve the *inner conflict*. In a drama
with a positive ending, the *outer action* resolves the *inner
conflict*. If action fails to resolve the inner conflict, the movie
qualifies as a tragedy. Your conflict is this: the person you
love is the person who is now responsible for your misery.
Your Beloved is your executioner! Recovery consists in
finding the proper action to resolve the inner conflict; it is
a heroic endeavor because heartbreak is an experience of
powerlessness and that is what every hero does: overcome
powerlessness. The psychological opposite of heroism is
victimization, which is to say that an unhealed heartbreak

turns you into a life-long victim. Losing your partner is sad enough; if you also turn yourself into a victim, it turns your drama into a tragedy.

Mourning, heartbreak, grief: same recovery

There are obvious differences between mourning the loss of somebody who dies, which is not a personal affront to you, and mourning the loss of somebody who *chooses* to leave you. The purpose of this book is not to look at the differences between these two kinds of heartbreak, but to help both the abandonee and the mourner begin a process of recovery, which is similar in both cases. I will be using, almost exclusively, examples where the abandonment is the result of a rejection by the partner because such an insult to the ego is best at uncovering the projections going on in love, more so even than when the partner dies. There is something final and tragic about losing your partner to death, yet there is something equally final and tragic in the recognition that one cannot resurrect the dead love of the abandoner. If you have been rejected, betrayed and abandoned, one of the best fantasies to entertain is to think of the abandoner as *dead*. It protects you against being hooked on the wrong kind of hope. We shall see later cases where the partners do get together after breakup, but in every case, it was possible only after a radical transformation of the relationship that lead to the breakup. Something has to die before you can reconnect with the abandoner and you have to mourn the relationship that existed prior to the breakup. If you partner just left, you may consider yourself just like a widow or widower, because you will have to follow the same steps to recovery. Conversely, if you are a widow or widower, consider yourself just like any other brokenhearted person; you too have to choose between stagnation or transformation, heroism or victimization. You too feel abandoned, betrayed and left out in the cold. The partner may not have wanted to die, but he/she did, and abandoned you in the misery of widowhood; you are now part of the same clan as all the other heartbroken individuals, with the same challenges, including the terrible blow to your ego. A partner abandoning you is one form dying can take, and a partner dying is one form abandonment can take. The cause for the abandonment is different, but the shock to the heart is similar, and the healing process the same. I use interchangeably the words bereavement, heartbreak, grief, mourning, loss, and abandonment, to describe the emotions of the person whose partner has left or died.

Widows and widowers often express how they regret not appreciating their partner more while he/she was still alive, confirming the popular wisdom that says "we don't know what we've got till it's gone." Having lost the other, the negative is often forgotten and memory wants to retain only the golden moments. It is a natural and beautiful way of preserving the best and discarding the worst. Nevertheless, this embellishment is possible only because the relationship has no more reality. Idealization provokes a fixation of the libido on to a non-existing love object. Now that the Beloved is absent, it is easy to project perfection on to the past relationship, like an orphan child who likes to imagine the absent parents as royalty. Part of your victimization comes from that dream of a perfection that never really existed. When your past love is sentimentalized and romanticized to the point of non-reality, it is not the greatness of love that is revealed, but your narcissistic wounding. It is as if you were saying "I don't care who he/she really was, I just want to remember a perfect love object who fulfilled my needs." Life is diminished when reality is forced to compete with the ghost of a perfect partner that never existed and can never exist because there are no perfect relationships. Over-sentimentalized relationships are a good indication that our narcissistic roots need trimming. Being abandoned inevitably provokes a narcissistic wounding and idealization is a normal defense mechanism against despair; yet, you need to move beyond your wounded ego. The dead partner may have been a most extraordinary human being, but the new reality is that you are now utterly abandoned in what, at first, feels like a hostile world. A process of *detachment* from the godlike figure of your absent partner is essential to the continuation of your emotional life. New persons become lovable only if the earlier loss has been properly mourned.

In some cases, the psychological process of mourning is already completed when the separation actually happens. Death or divorce can mark the final expression of a long, often unconscious detachment, especially when a long sickness, or a long solitary marriage gave you time to adapt to a reality in which the partner is absent. In those cases the transition to a new relationship can happen very quickly. Nevertheless, it is a well-known fact that moving too quickly or too *unconsciously* to a new commitment can signal the repetition of the same neurotic pattern over and over again. Those who hold onto the naive belief that the next partner will finally, at last, be the magical Lover, the one with the power to resolve all the conflicts, both inner and outer, often go in rapid succession from one partner to the next, repeating the same neurotic form of attachment that leads to failure. Certainly, after a heartbreak, a new relationship is longed for, and sometimes a transitional affair (band-aid lover, friend with benefits) may help the long term transition, but only if one is aware that the energy is still bound to the previous relationship until the mourning is over. Psychologists of all schools agree that failure to examine the ingrained primitive affects involved in heartbreak may lead to the deterioration of the capacity to love. Unhealed heartbreaks can bring on the fate that is most feared: isolation in a loveless world.

Medical research confirms that heartbreak is a very serious health hazard and should not be left to fester in the unconscious. Beneath various symptoms of depression and anxiety, one finds an un-mourned loss, a loss that the patient keeps recreating in all adult relationships. Again, it is a situation where one either jumps one rung on the ladder of evolution or suffers stagnation, regression, deterioration. A heartbroken person is just like a refugee, a displaced person, having to orient himself in a new emotional environment.

The challenge is very difficult and very dangerous: those who fail shrivel, both psychically and physically. Those who survive do so because they create a post-heartbreak identity. The message from neuroscience is clear: following the trauma of heartbreak, you either evolve or you deteriorate; it is the *use it or lose it* theory of neuroplasticity, a kind of scientific confirmation that when you find yourself in deep waters, either you sink or you swim. This book wants to be a swimming lesson, with perhaps a session or two on the high board. As a teenager, I was trained as swimming instructor and earned pocket money giving private swimming lessons in the summer. The first and most challenging student I ever had was a friend of my parents, a philosopher and professor of formal logic. At 60, he was still very afraid of water but ready to trust the fifteen-year-old girl I was then, because of the Red Cross Instructor Badge sewn on my swimming suit. I began the lessons in immersion, following the principles I had learned, to acquire my precious badge. He resisted going underwater and wanted me to go on *explaining* all about the experience of being underwater: how it would feel, if he would still be able to see underwater and how exactly would he surmount the terror of going under. Before plunging in, he wanted complete intellectual understanding of the process that would prevent him from choking. After exhausting all my repertoire of metaphors to *explain* the process, I finally grabbed him by the shoulders, and, one…two… three… pinch your nose professor… I am now pulling you under. He had no choice but to follow. Resurfacing, he was absolutely delighted, and his facial expression was like that of a five year old discovering the pleasure of playing in the water. He had conquered his lifelong fear of water. That is what grief did to me: it pulled me under, except that there was no lifeguard, no swimming instructor, no reassurance. After almost drowning in tears, I emerged with a sense of having surmounted some of my lifelong terrors and with a changed perspective on love and relationships. Now I want to share the recovery and the discoveries.

I am not a believer in miracles, quick easy cures, ready made formulas and motivational pep talks to convince you to *move on*. Finding the way out is a bit more complicated than that, because it is a *learning process* to change the wiring of the brain. Learning is a process that engages the intellect as well as the emotions, which is the reason I am presenting the scientific evidence, to engage you *intellectually* in understanding the physiological dimensions of a loss of love. I have also experienced first hand the absolute necessity of immersion in the riches of the arts and the humanities, to engage the emotions and keep the heart open. When it comes to healing, stories are as important as theories. Daniel Siegel (2007, 2009, 2009) who coined the term *Interpersonal Neurobiology* demonstrates the importance of stories to coordinate right and left hemispheres. His work supports what Jungians have known for a very long time—that the formulation of a narrative, the reading, recitation and sharing of other's stories, and the telling of dreams makes a difference in the healing process. As there will be quite a bit of neuroscientific explanations in this book, I want to add the flavor of literature, and ground the process of recovery in as full a narrative as possible. In order to do that, this first chapter opens with a narrative: the story of William. It is *not* a clinical case history, in the sense that William's story was *not* written from the outside by a psychologist observing the patient, *not* written in the clinical language of the Diagnostic Statistical Manual and it is *not* meant as anecdotal evidence. The function of all the vignettes through this book is to *illustrate and inspire,* as stories are supposed to do. It goes without saying that each story of grief is different; that everyone reacts with their own personality; that the resolution sometimes takes weeks and sometimes years; that heartbreaks have different causes and different outcomes. Yet, they all have the same archetypal core because heartbroken individuals all suffer the same kind of torture. It is this archetypal core that I wish to outline by telling you stories based in reality and written in collaboration with the person recovering from heartbreak.

William is a man of fifty-two, a tenured professor of geography, studying for a second Ph.D. in psychology. I first met him as my student in the Ph.D. program where I teach. We later became friends. To cross the desert of heartbreak and come out psychically alive and physically healthy takes courage and William happens to be emotionally brave. He was willing to contribute his story for this book under the same agreement I have with all the others whose stories I use throughout this book. Our agreement was that he would talk about his grief—many hours—and I would translate those emotions in a short written narrative—many versions— until we both felt my words matched his experience. I appreciated working with him because he had enough maturity to accept that the mischievous god of love likes to make fun of our standards of normality when it comes to love-struck humans. William is not ashamed of having made a fool of himself and telling me all about this *love madness*. His story is the ordinary story of an ordinary heartbreak happening to an average, so called normal and functioning individual. In other words, his story is typical, no... the right word again is *archetypal* because beyond the idiosyncrasies, his experience exemplifies the profound emotions of all heartbreaks. An archetypal story is like a basic melody: whatever variations you may add, however you mix and arrange the score, you can still recognize the melody. Hearing the first four notes of Beethoven's ninth symphony on someone's iPhone is enough to identify the whole complex symphony. The melody of heartbreak is similar: it is a timeless and universal score in which you can recognize the basic emotions, regardless of the individual variations.

William was married once, for fifteen years, a good-enough marriage although not a passionate one. His first marriage ended without drama, with both he and his wife agreeing to a shared responsibility for their three adolescent daughters. William then fell passionately in love with Laura, ten years younger and with no children of her own. Right from the beginning of that relationship William made it clear to Laura that he was not willing nor able to start a second family because he had chosen sterilization as a means of contraception after fathering his three daughters. William also expressed, from the start, his views about the traditional institution of marriage and his dislike of its contractual nature. Although he valued monogamy and fidelity, and although he was helping Laura financially at times when she was unemployed, he did not wish to legalize their relationship. Laura, initially, seemed fine with William's values; she herself did not want children and did not care much for the traditional marriage vows. Yet, she soon resented the fact that she was not the unique focus of William's love and attention; she was regularly distressed by William's close connection to his three daughters, by William's travels and studies, by William's numerous friends, including his ex-wife.

I began taking notes about William's story at the time he discovered that Laura was having an affair. At first, the cool denial of his obvious panic reminded me of what a policeman once told me: victims of a car crash, in a state of shock, often act a bit too cool. Women typically worry about locating their purse while men ask about the damages to their car. Only later does it come to their mind that they are hurt and then they start shivering and taking in the reality of the situation. William, in the initial phase of his heartbreak, showed the same bland reaction that indicates what, in psychology, we call denial. True to the definition of a *defense mechanism*, denial protected him for a while: he talked about Laura's betrayal as if it was just a little bump in the road, certain he could fix it by being generous and understanding with the betrayer.

DENIAL: THIS CAN'T BE!

When I met Laura, it was the first time in my life that I believed in destiny. I still think Laura is my soulmate, we are destined for each other. I received from her everything that I came on this earth to receive. From the beginning, she said that I was the great love of her life, that ours was the most profound emotional and sexual relationship she had ever had. Since our very first moments of intimacy, four years ago, I have felt that particular form of contentment that gives love its glorious reputation.

I knew last night, for sure, that Laura was having an affair with someone she must have met during the two weeks of her trip to Europe. She and I have such a deep connection, I felt something was off the minute I picked her up at the airport. I was eager to reconnect and that evening, I wanted to make love to her. Although we went through the motions of lovemaking, she was not present to "us": she was aloof. That was Friday evening. The whole weekend was bizarre; Laura was nice but silent, sweet in a cold distant sort of way. On Monday, when she left for work, my first thought was that she had met someone on that business trip to London, after which she had taken a week off to visit Paris. I could not help committing the indiscretion of opening her computer and reading her emails. She must have forgotten that I had the password, or maybe she just could not imagine how revealing was her sudden sexual withdrawal.

The emails revealed it all: my rival is Jack, whom I know, because we both train at the same gym. I read the email she sent him last night, when I was in the shower, just before we made love. I also read the one she sent this morning before leaving for work. I read the ones they exchanged before leaving on that trip and I saw the pictures of their romance in London and Paris. Laura writes that she now envisions, with Jack, "a long life of love, travel, loyalty and rich conversations." Jack writes back that he feels certain Laura is the woman he has been waiting for, all his life.

How can they both be that naïve? Certitude and promises of eternal love after a brief romantic escapade? Come on! How can Laura confuse an affair with the kind of deep soul connection that is ours? Laura's betrayal baffles me, her naiveté disappoints me; doesn't she know that a summer fling is not on the same level as a soul mate? I can forgive an affair; it is not a pleasant thing, but affairs happen. For now, she is acting like an hormone-driven, love-struck silly teenager but I am convinced it will pass. I think Laura is having this affair to get even with me: she does not like the friendship I have with my ex-wife, it makes her feel insecure. Since our divorce, my ex and I never had any kind of sexual connection, but still Laura resents that we remained friends. And I know she resents the attention I give to my three adolescent daughters. Laura would like to be the center of my universe and when my daughters are around, it makes her feel unimportant.

I supported Laura through periods of unemployment, lack of resources; I have been on her side, proving my love with acts of love, not just words. And now, she falls for Jack's sweet promises? I want to shake her up, to wake her up from her girlish illusions. I know Jack. He is indeed a nice guy, but he too has a history. Jack is the father of a three year old baby boy. For now, that baby is just a sweet little creature, and Laura writes about this baby as if it was a cute house-pet. She has no idea how an adorable baby eventually turns into an impossible teen, like my girls now are.

Laura is so smitten by Jack, she won't even discuss the possibility that her affair is a sweet delusion. I can't believe Laura believes Jack's promises to deliver a lifetime of sweet love and good conversation as if a honeymoon could go on forever. I can't recognize Laura in that naïve woman, but I trust she'll wake up from her delusion. I know that somebody in a love infatuation won't hear the voice of reason. I am patient. She'll come to see that my love is truer than Jack's. She is too much in her pink bubble right now to even engage in a meaningful conversation with me.

All the while my internal dialogue with her doesn't stop. I am having a one way, silent argument with her and with the world. "Laura, Laura, don't you see that you and I belong to each other for all eternity? Don't you see I am more worthy of your love than Jack will ever be?"

When one partner has an affair, the outsider —or predator, in this case, Jack— seems to offer precisely what is missing. Although Laura does love William, she resents many things: his three daughters, his friendship with his ex-wife, his busy social life, his numerous friends; all that threatens Laura's sense of a secure attachment. By contrast, Jack makes her feel that she is the *one and only*, the center of his universe. Jack's baby boy has little reality for Laura because he is with his mother most of the time.

In the following weeks Laura keeps herself so busy that William's attempts at reconnecting don't get past her busyness. She won't tell William that it's over nor will she discuss their future. She blames her work schedule, the crisis in her family (her mother is sick, her sister is divorcing, her brother lost his job…). If Laura keeps William on a hook, it is not out of malice or manipulation, but because the betrayer and the betrayed can both be in denial. William won't consider that the relationship might be over, while Laura won't face the fact that she is destroying the relationship that, as she used to tell William, has been the most profound in her life.

The next phase for William is what a clinician would describe as a *maniacal episode*, again a typical reaction to the initial shock of heartbreak.

EMAIL OBSESSION

Laura has moved out of my house; she rented her own apartment to "sort out her feelings." I know it is because she wants to be with Jack. I check my emails obsessively, longing, deprived, sad, depressed, filled with the hope that this sorting out of her feelings will end with a sweet contrite email: "Jack is a big mistake, it's you I love, I am coming home." I can't even go the grocery store without thinking I might miss her call, her visit.

When we do get together, Laura is aloof, physically impermeable to my gestures of affection. I fear Laura is choosing Jack over me and it sends me into a panic. Each time I panic, I send her another email. Every day, I spend hours crafting long eloquent pleas, and Laura answers back with falsely sweet and short replies like : "Thanks for your lovely email; I am processing so much right now, please give me time and space. I hope you are taking good care of your precious self." My hopes are raised when she writes sweet words and I send more long and affectionate messages. Sometimes she takes two or three days before she answers back an uncompromising brief reply: "I love you too! I am so busy right now, I can't reply properly but I'll see you next week." She cancels our meetings one time out of two, always with a good reason. I am hooked on our email connection like an umbilical cord that attaches me to life. It is torture.

William can't let go of his hope, a hope that is his worst enemy. Hope makes him live in the future, but detachment can only happen in the present. Hope makes William strategize obsessively, firing one email after another— a typical maniacal behavior. The psychosomatic consequences of such mania begin to add up. The body always carries what the psyche refuses to acknowledge and William soon shows symptoms of heart arrythmia (irregular heartbeat). He feels caught in a labyrinth, a universal symbol for the emotional disorientation of grief. In a labyrinth, every path leads to a dead end. William's dead end is a belief: that the return of the partner is the only way out of his misery. If you are hooked on hope, feeling as if in a labyrinth, obsessing and strategizing like a rat in the labyrinth, it indicates that you are still in shock. It may look like this:

THE RAT IN THE LABYRINTH

For the past two months, I have been feeling like a rat in a labyrinth trying every trick to get the food pellets and not getting any. Laura insists that she still loves me, although she admits that she is also very much attracted to Jack. At least she is honest, and does not deny seeing Jack.

I keep telling her that infidelity and affairs do happen and don't necessarily mean the end of our relationship. I keep asking her: do you have the motivation, the desire, the strength, to continue this difficult voyage WITH ME? Or are you choosing a different road, a life with Jack? She can't answer, she is ambivalent. I beg her to come back home because I still have confidence that, together, because of our profound connection, we could navigate through this dark sea. I despair when I feel that she boarded Jack's ship! I don't want her to protect me against the truth and tell me sweet lies, like when she says she is busy with work and I know she is busy with Jack. What I need more than anything is the truth, not another layer of padding with her sweet lies. Laura is sweet but not courageous when it comes to telling things as they are. Her covertness, her aloofness make me crazy.

We spent the last weekend together, at my house, because I begged her to come. She accepted, probably because it was Jack's monthly weekend with his infant son. She spent most of our Saturday on the phone with her mom and her sister, then she washed her car (whom she treats with more tenderness than she cares to give me), then she groomed her cat (who follows her everywhere she goes) then she went to the veterinarian with her cat because it had an eye infection. When we finally got to bed on Saturday evening, she could claim exhaustion to fall asleep the minute her head hit the pillow. Laura is an athletic runner, and on Sunday morning, right after coffee, she ran a good four miles. While my heart sinks, bleeds, she runs, she sleeps, she talks on the phone, writes emails, takes care of her cat, her car, her fitness. Why do I still care about her? On days like this, I find we have little in common. What is the mystery of my attachment to her? Laura says she is being true to her soul by exploring her attraction to Jack; that she has to follow her instinct and her instinct tells her to put a hold on the incredibly strong sexual bond that used to unite us body and soul. How can I contradict her instinct? What is it that I don't get? She does not seem to be conscious that she is breaking my heart. I am in deep mourning of what used to be, but she doesn't seem very concerned. She tortures me with her sexless gentleness! I am ten years older than both Laura and Jack. Is that why I am slower to detach? Am I too old for love? Finished? I wonder how she could have felt our love as the greatest of her life and then, poof! gone, evaporated, and Jack is her new God. Does Laura even realize the amount of destruction that comes from severing our sexual connection? How innocent can a forty year old woman be? I am profoundly ashamed of my clinging to Laura, because I suspect that I refuse to look at the obvious: Laura 's love has migrated. I feel surges of revolt and rebellion.

After running another three miles on Sunday afternoon, she showered and we sat outside on the patio to watch sunset. It was just Laura and I again, looking at the golden light in the garden, drinking a glass of white wine, my heart ready to forgive and forget her affair with Jack, just peace and joy again. I was certain we were reconnecting and would make love that night, the crystalline purity of our connection dispelling all the fog of her betrayal. Then her cell phone rang, she took the call, her embarrassment so obvious. She said her woman friend needed her to come by. It was so obviously a lie, it actually embarrassed me. Of course Jack wanted her to come to his place; his infant son safely returned to his mom, he was ready for Laura to visit. My distress peaked like sudden fever. This arrow got me at the core. I spent the night sweating, my heart jumping in its cage like a scared cat caught in a net.

From then on I have remained in a daze, slow

to feel, slow to think, hobbling haltingly from one necessary task to another, but with a heart beating too fast. I get food, eat food, digest food. I wash dishes, do my work, put my body to bed, and obliterate every thought or feeling. I am slowly progressing toward emotional catatonia. I feel a weariness of every organ, a misery of the oldest kind, I guess you would call it the death wish, or maybe love-sickness, because it does feel like a sickness, depleting me of energy.

My imagination is stuck in the hope of receiving even a crumb of love from Laura the Good Girl with the deaf/mute heart! I am trying, as my friends advise me, to "take care of myself." For now, it feels impossible! There is only one person in the whole world who can take care of me: Laura, and I have lost access to that person.

What is Love? I don't know anymore; I am utterly confused. I used to believe human love was the highest form of spirituality, and now it feels like the cruelest lie. I have experienced love as a great spasm of pleasure, an exclamation of joy, a physical and spiritual high, and now the love in my heart feels like a tumor, a cancerous growth, a force that keeps me in bondage. If love is not bondage, how can I explain that, after six months of her coldness, I am still, against all hope, waiting for Laura to express sexual desire for me?

The dark side of love

William's experience of the dark side of love belongs to the very nature of the sentiment; we are all agnostic (i.e. unknowing) when it comes to the mysterious nature of love. How could we not? Of all times, love has been symbolized by many things and their opposites: a cradle and a coffin; an initiation and a blinding; a lotus blooming in the heart, and an arrow piercing it; a school of mystery and a torture; a spiritual discipline, a sport, an entertainment, a game, a war, a form of hygiene, a divine rapture. It has been said that human love is pure/dirty, angelic/diabolical, divine/evil. It is described as the most intense *physical* experience, the basic *psychological* experience, the most *spiritual* experience. It is felt as a blessing and a curse, a remedy and a sickness, a pair of handcuffs and a pair of wings, a glorious aura and a rope around the neck, an elevation of the heart and a falling down. William feels all the contradictory symbols of love, *which is the truth of love*. His confusion is legitimate, it is what Jung called the tension of the opposites, which is what propels us to individuate. As that tension keeps mounting, so does his panic. His psychosomatic state is now much worse than when he first discovered Laura's betrayal. This is the point where William is most love-crazy, as if nature was pushing him to make an *evolutionary jump*.

Here is somebody who is usually a fully functioning man, a rational person, a professor of geography who just defended a second Ph.D. in psychology. He is not a young naïve lover, not a beginner, not a pathological co-dependent.

Before his marriage to the mother of his daughters, William had been involved with four other women, with whom he had had strong erotic connections, which eventually faded and turned into friendships. After his divorce, he remained a responsible father for his three daughters, even as he began the passionate relationship to Laura. Until the breakup with Laura, William had always been the one to terminate a relationship. The erotic attraction to Laura was the most intense of all his relationships, the heat of his passion amplifying all his unconscious needs and fears. With the loss of that connection, William began to turn inward, to *introvert,* to use a Jungian expression. With the help of a therapist, he started uncovering the unconscious threat that makes him so fearful of Laura's aloofness and ambivalence. He discovered a primitive, pre-verbal experience of having been neglected by his socially prominent mother, a rather cold woman. His ancient terror could only resurface if a woman turned cold on him, as did Laura, as opposed to all his previous relationships, where he was the abandoner. Laura taking her distance reactivated William's unbearable vulnerability as a child, a situation he had learned to avoid with *all* woman, except, of course, the first time, with his mother. I am tempted to say that Laura's natural ambivalence and aloofness is precisely what *attracted* him, *so he could have his heart broken*, and evolve past the ancient fear. The psyche is naturally oriented toward the past (mom and dad and the past traumas…) but it is as naturally oriented toward the future[1], provoking what needs to happen for the next chapter to unfold. The unconscious fear may be different for each person, yet, the lesson to learn is the same for everyone: "you are an adult now, and you are not as vulnerable as you were as a child." Laura too is acting from her own primitive fear, not only William. Laura has repeatedly expressed to William her fear of not being *enough,* as she had felt in her family of origin. When she had the affair with Jack, he seemed to promise exclusive devotion to Laura, as opposed to William complex network of familial, professional and friendly relations that made her feel that she was not the *one and only.* Laura was ready to believe that Jack's exclusive attention could free her from her fear of not being enough. From then on, Laura and William entered a dance that Beethoven's music expresses so well: the beauty of love, the chaos of fear. All relationships contain a measure of unconscious tangles; unraveling the threads is part of life's adventure. Both Laura and William are locked in unconscious, *pre-verbal, implicit memories* that make them hurt each other like two animals in a cage.

For the next couple of months, William and Laura remain in this intense emotional dance, where the unconscious attraction toward reunion is a strong as the unconscious fear of reunion. They still see each other from time to time, they email and they talk over the phone. Although William is always asking for a clarification of their relationship, Laura is incapable of closure, keeping William hooked on hope. One morning, William receives registered mail for Laura and he tries to reach her to tell her to come get her mail.

Receiving no answer for four days, he becomes worried and comes unannounced to her apartment, early in the morning, with the intention of giving her the mail before she leaves for work. Laura's apartment is a little studio built on top of the double garage of a large property, and the staircase that leads to her entrance door offers a view on her bedroom window. William comes up the stairs, the blinds of the bedroom window are not completely drawn, and peeking through the window, he sees Jack soundly asleep beside Laura. There is a bunch of open suitcases and boxes all over the bedroom floor, indicating that Jack has moved in with Laura, a scene he had not anticipated. Laura hears the sound of William climbing the stairs and sees him staring through the window. She comes to the front door, steps out on the porch, and closes the door behind her, reacting with hostility to what she feels is an intrusion. The situation, as she later explains to William, reminded her of her intrusive and controlling mother. Her hostile reaction stupefies William, and constitutes the turning point, one that happens in all heartbreaks, the point where you either detach or get very sick.

DETACH OR DIE

I shall remember that morning all my life; she came out and stood barefoot on the porch, barring the door as if I might have the intention of forcing my way in. I was so obviously far from any intention of intruding that I was bewildered by her hostility. She had not informed me that Jack was moving in with her and there he was, moving in, suitcases and all. I was shivering from head to toe, feeling how she had lied to me, a lie by omission, but a lie nevertheless. My heartbeat was out of control, I was breathless, and my mouth was so dry I could barely pronounce words; I was just there, shivering, silent and broken. Laura was emotionally cold, shut down, unaware that I was about to faint. She called my presence an "intrusion on her privacy, a crossing of her psychic boundaries." That was the language she had used many times to talk about her intrusive mother and her abusive father. Indeed, both her parents had repeatedly "intruded in her privacy," and "crossed her psychic boundaries" in ways that anybody would qualify as abusive. But I had come out of concern for her, unaware the Jack had moved in. I had knocked on the door, I did not break in. That cold hostile person in front of me was not the Laura I thought I knew, but the rebellious teenager, the very girl she had described to me so many times, angry and obliged to defend her autonomy against a controlling mother and an irresponsible aloof father. That Laura was not my equal, not my friend, not somebody who could understand the vulnerable state I was in. She was the fragile angry adolescent girl, afraid of having been caught in a deceit, incapable of seeing that I was somebody about to collapse on the floor. She asked me to "leave the premises immediately," but I was in no state to drive. I was having a panic attack, my heart racing like crazy. I begged her to come sit with me in my car parked in her driveway, until my heartbeat went back to normal. I don't remember, in my whole life, ever begging for a woman's compassion like I did that morning. I was five years old again, imploring my mother for help because I was burning with a 104 degree fever and thought I was dying. The coldness in Laura's eyes was just like the coldness in my mother's face when I disturbed one of her social events because I was sick, or needed something for class, or had to ask her for something, anything... Laura's lack of compassion for my obvious physical distress went through me like a sword.

She agreed curtly to follow me to my car and sat with me as if she had no other choice but to placate a needy child. After a few minutes she expressed again that I should "respect her privacy" and "leave the premises" so she could go back inside and have her breakfast with Jack! She repeated again that my visit was an "assault on her privacy" and that she did not owe me any explanation about her new situation with Jack. I left. Maybe there was indeed a semi-

conscious need in me to check if Jack had moved in with her; if so, isn't it legitimate to want to uncover a truth I was beginning to intuit? Hadn't she been lying in my face for the past six months? But my most troubling emotion was not the experience of her utter lack of compassion, and of having been deceived, it was an uncanny physical sensation. I felt cast in the role of her intrusive parents and at the same time I was regressing to my own infantile distress. She was reacting to her parents, not to the shivering, vulnerable and defeated ex-lover in front of her. She was not with me, not in our story, she was reacting to her past! I had suddenly become her controlling mother, who controlled the way she dressed, the friends she had, the way she voted, the books she read, the places she went. Laura was reacting as well to her insensitive egocentric father, one who did not protect her against the intrusiveness and control of the mother. I was not there as me, William, I was both the father and the mother who wounded her. The same is true of me: I was not reacting to a woman caught in a lie, but to my own withdrawn mother. I too was reacting to a past I had never confronted.

That experience was defining for me; it created a "before" and an "after." Before this episode I was confident that Laura and I could get over the crisis of

*her affair with Jack. After, there was no more "us,"
no more "we." I was hurting, but it was now clear
that I was hurting alone and that I was hurting from
more than Laura's betrayal. I was hurting from my
own unconscious wounds, my unfinished business
with my past, my immature expectations about love
(eternal... perfect... all giving... healing...). I began
detaching, the Laura-and-I couple was finally dead,
and I, a widower like so many others who have lost
their spouse.*

[handwritten: Not only Sexual betrayal but pain for past wounds]

Relationships are complicated, and infidelity often
destroys them, but, contrary to the dominant moral
discourse, it is not necessarily the sexual nature of betrayal
that fractures the connection. It is crucial to examine
what, exactly, breaks the heart. The tendency, in many a
psychological theory, has been to emphasize the sexual
aspect of betrayal, which perpetuates biased theories about
relationships. William's traumatic experience is *not only* a
reaction to the sexual connotation of seeing Laura in bed
with Jack; he already knew about Laura's affair with Jack.
The real turning point was the shock that delivered a major
insight: Laura's aloofness brought to his awareness his fear
of his own mother's aloofness. Both Laura and William
were reacting to the past: she to abusive parents, and he to
a mother who could suddenly give him the cold shoulder,

[handwritten: If you were Simon to do important!]

unresponsive to his distress. He suddenly *saw* how the panic in him was the reactivation of the unconscious alarm from the past as if his brain were saying: "ALERT! here is a cold, detached, uncaring woman like your mother." This is the peak: a bumping against the pre-verbal synaptic bundles that contain the deadly threat of abandonment for a dependent infant.

Before telling the next phase of William's recovery, lets us make a detour through the territory of neuroscience to understand that basic unavoidable sense of alarm that happens when experiencing loss of love. The next chapter summarizes, from a neurological point of view, what makes love so necessary and so volatile and why a rejection from the partner can make you act so irrationally. It is important to understand *why* mourning and lovesickness can lead to psychotic breaks, murderous behaviors, panic attacks and heart pain similar to a heart attack. The more you know about what causes your brain to become dysfunctional, the more you can search for what can support its recovery. You need to understand how *psychological* insights can modify the neural network that transmits your thoughts and feelings and how becoming more conscious of your emotions can create adaptive behaviors. For those psychological insights to happen, it is useful to start with a *rational* (scientific) understanding of that most *irrational* experience: love. Let's look at what part of the brain is reacting to what, why, and how. A scientific understanding is helpful before one can dive into the psychological depths, where personal meaning is to be found. Although it is true that the resolution of a heartbreak asks for something more than scientific explanations, something more than medication to calm the panic, it remains extremely useful to have a scientific understanding of our symptoms of love-sickness. Recovery is a re-wiring of both the left and right hemispheres of the brain. Neuroscience can explain why it is so and where in the brain it is happening but it cannot, by itself, make it happen. For the reconstruction of your self, you need to fish at a deeper level; this is where a depth psychological approach becomes necessary. But before we get to the depth psychological perspective, let's review the neurological perspective.

CHAPTER 2

THE THREE CHARACTERS IN
THE NEUROLOGICAL DRAMA

> *As far as happiness is concerned, its main utility is to make unhappiness possible. We need to form loving and trusting relationships for their rupture to cause us the precious wrenching we call unhappiness. Without the experience of happiness, or even the hope of it, unhappiness would not be so cruel, and as a consequence, would not bear fruits.*
>
> Marcel Proust[9]

> *Trust and the possibility of betrayal come into the world at the same moment...and betrayal, as a continual possibility to be lived with, belongs to trust just as doubt belongs to a living faith.*
>
> James Hillman[10]

One of the first widely disseminated theories about the brain is probably that of Paul MacLean, who in 1952 suggested that the brain is really three brains in one, each the result of a distinct stage of evolution: the reptilian brain, the limbic (or mammalian) brain, and the human neocortex; hence the name *triune theory of the brain*. This theory can help us understand why the above quotations make sense, and how the pain of heartbreak can be a factor of evolution, a real push from nature to force us to evolve past the level of purely animal reactions.

MacLean's theory has been and still is extremely popular, in education, psychology, and psychiatry, as well as in popular scientific magazines. It became popular for a good reason: it was one of the first to explain our most irrational behavior, such as the love-madness that accompanies heartbreak. Thomas Insels, director of the National Institute of Mental Health in Rockville, summarizes the argument about the enduring validity of MacLean's theory when he points out that, although MacLean's triune theory of the brain is past its utility for ultra-specialized research in the lab, it has opened the door for neuroscience to ask *big philosophical questions* about love, consciousness and freedom, instead of the more tractable questions about vision and movement in frogs catching flies and rats becoming depressed when separated from the mother[11]. Those *big* questions are the ones that the heartbroken person needs to entertain, not the ultra-specialized ones about brain functions. One does not need to be a neuroscientist to grasp the still valid core of MacLean's model, which is the idea that some brain structures, and their associated behaviors, are the result of evolution, similar to what Jung called the *million year old psyche*. In plain words, it means we have no choice but to deal with the primitive person in us that makes its presence felt when there is a loss of love.

I will use a literary device dear to archetypal psychology: personification of abstract notions, or, as James Hillman likes to call this method: a personnifying[12]. It allows me to organize the scientific information in the form of a narrative with three main characters: imagine your brain as a stage, on which the *crude crocodile*, the *puny puppy* and the *wise human* are playing out their conflict. Like a computer Identity Game, your fate depends on which of those three characters takes control of your mind/brain. The victory of the wise human defines the positive outcome — in which winning equals healing— but this character can't win if you ignore the other two actors in your drama. Let us introduce each of the three characters, as well as the neurological reality they symbolize.

1) The crude crocodile (reptilian brain): "I don't know what got into me when I shot her"

This part of the brain is called reptilian because we share it with crocodiles, lizards, and other reptiles. It comprises the spinal cord, the brainstem, the diencephalon and the basal ganglia; it is responsible for our basic reflexes (fight or flight), for breathing, swallowing, heartbeat, startle reflex, and the visual tracking systems. The primitiveness of the reptilian brain tragically shows up everyday in court rooms: a jealous lover coldly kills the rival and then says, "When

I found out that she betrayed me with this guy, I was blind with rage, possessed, I don't know what got into me" —a typical reaction from the reptilian brain. This demonstrates the persistence of a primitive set of reactions in *all* of us, which is why we can empathize with Othello's rage. Many individuals are serving life sentences, or live under restraining orders, because of their incapacity to understand and evolve beyond their crocodile psychology. A heartbreak *necessarily* activates those primitive reactions and, as with all reflexes, they are absolutely uncontrollable by the conscious will. However, although no one has control of the immediate *surge* of an impulse, we do have control of the *behavior* that follows the first crocodile reflex. Those who don't may end up in prison!

What neuroscience teaches us here is crucial: we cannot *control* our brain, we can only *relate* to it. *Relating* to the crocodile (the reflex impulse in the brain) means we must first *acknowledge* the urge to hurt or kill the rival. Only then can we use the higher functions of the brain to avoid *acting on the impulse*. This is called self-control, or self-regulation of affect, or self-discipline. Normally, we begin learning affect regulation in infancy, when mom urges us to think before we act! In this *relating* is our chance to change the pattern of neuronal response.

A good example of this two-step process of relating to the crocodile is given by the Buddhist monk who develops an above-average capacity to *relate* to the events happening in his brain. Faced with an instinctual threat—a scorpion in his shoe, a snake in his path, a racing car about to hit him—his brain, just like anybody's brain, responds with the ultra-quick *startle reflex* that is the result of the activation of the reptilian brain. Just as the crocodile snoozing on the beach becomes instantly awake when it senses the slightest movement on the ground, the monk is startled. This startle reflex is faster than the emotion of fear, because fear is located in the limbic brain (our actor number two in the drama) and fear is a bit too slow to register, as compared to the ultra-quick reptilian avoidance reflex. A crocodile, who does not have a limbic brain, does not *feel* what we call fear; it reacts with the same reflex as a frog catching a fly, a cobra striking at its prey. The reptilian reaction is fast and focused, but with no feeling tone. Humans possess this most primitive level of reflex, which we need for survival. At birth, we check reflexes to confirm the proper functioning of this primitive part of the brain. The monk reacts with that same instinctual alert, but the difference from the average untrained person is the amount of time it will take for homeostasis to come back and calm down. The trained monk does not *control* his reflexes more than you and I do, but he *relates* differently to the other parts of his brain. When faced with a speeding car about to hit, one should put the brakes on without having to think about it; the reptilian reflex is the most competent in this situation. The reaction of limbic fear, one that we share with mammals, comes a millisecond later. The difference between the trained monk's reaction and mine consists in the monk's capacity to prevent the reptilian reflex from flooding the whole limbic circuitry. A trained brain has to *relate* to the crocodile brain; the monk does put the brakes on without having to think about it, yet his training helps him limit the next stage of reaction, which is the limbic emotion of fear and anger at the offensive driver. A heartbreak is the perfect occasion to learn the monk's trick, and not end up in prison because you pulled the trigger without thinking.

Imagine a woman comfortably seated in a cinema; she is relaxed, watching a comedy. A man and a woman in the row in front of her are kissing. Suddenly she recognizes the man as her husband, and he is kissing another woman! Immediately all the systems regulated by the reptilian brain are on the alert mode—her respiration, blood circulation, heartbeat, body temperature, and perspiration begin responding to the threat just as if the theater was on fire. Popular language reflects this physiological reality: "When I saw them kiss, my heart stopped, my blood froze. I was white (or red, or blue) in the face. I choked. First I was shivering, then I was boiling with rage." These are all the alerts of the reptilian brain. Witnessing the betrayal creates an incredible amount of somatic disturbance in her autonomous nervous system, which is regulated by the reptilian brain. She will experience difficulty with digestion, sleep, heart rate, blood pressure, hormonal flow; her crocodile is acting out his part! Neuroscientists use the concept of *allostasis*, a word that means maintaining stability (stasis) through change (allo) and is often used as a synonym for the basic reptilian stress response. For example, the woman's breathing *has to* change and become heavier (allo) and her heart *has* to beat faster (allo) for her body to still get air into her lungs (stasis). In other words, her organism, in order to adapt to this traumatic event, has to maintain stability through change, even at great cost to her organism. The term "allostatic load" refers to the cumulative cost to the body when the extra effort is too much, or carried for too long, like the excessive wear and tear on a machine. An *acute* stress may actually stimulates the immune system and is a necessary strategy of the body to run away from danger, but a *chronic* stress shuts it down, the best example of which is what psychologists call a *burn-out*. The allostatic load of the woman witnessing her husband's betrayal starts with a form of *acute* stress (the emotional shock of betrayal); if she continues to react with a high level of alarm long after the incident in the cinema, it qualifies as *chronic* stress and creates somatic damage. Her husband's betrayal makes her literally sick because she keeps feeling it, with the same physiological responses.

A crocodile has a choice of only two instinctual responses: fight or flight. The crocodile bites if the enemy is chewable, and runs for cover if the enemy is too big to fight. The woman in the cinema produces the chemical cocktail that would allow her either to attack her husband, or to run out of the theater in a panic; yet because her brain offers more options than that of the crocodile, the second actor in the drama shows up and complicates the drama with emotional distress.

2) The wimpy-puny-puppy (mammalian brain)

Mammals possess a layer of brain over the crocodile:

the limbic brain, composed of the hippocampus, the amygdala, the hypothalamus and periventricular structures. Neuroscientists have recently demonstrated exactly how the amygdala makes animal emotions possible. The amygdala is an emotional alarm, the dispenser of the emotion of fear. It is also the keeper of a permanent implicit memory of every past situation, context, symbol, image, object, odor, sound, or personality type that has ever provoked that fear.[13] This primary level of feeling remains with us all our life. As Jill Bolte Taylor writes: "It is interesting to note that although our limbic system functions throughout our lifetime, it does not mature. As a result, when our emotional "buttons" are pushed, we retain the ability to react to incoming stimulation as though we were a two year old, even when we are adults."[14]

The whole limbic/emotional brain is responsible for a repertoire of reactions that are basically mammalian reactions. We shouldn't be too embarrassed by our wimpy begging for the partner to come back, as we are reacting just like a lost pup trying to attract the attention of the mother. One of the reasons we can get so attached to our pets is that they offer a good measure of what neuroscientists call "limbic regulation," a kind of bonding that exists between humans and between humans and their pets. Mammal's capacity for attachment also shows us, as in a mirror, our own need for affection, care, play, security, comfort. It also mirrors our acute distress at being separated from the source of protection and affection. This distress is the first innate manifestation of *anxiety*. The memory of those painful moments are without words (that is why they are called *pre-verbal*, or *implicit* memory), because they happened before the linguistic capacity is fully developed (around eighteen months of age in humans). Before the development of language, the words to tell ourselves the story are not there yet. The memory of all fearful events is inscribed in the limbic brain and comes back when the experience of abandonment is repeated in adult life[15]. That is how horses as well as kids remember not to pet a poisonous snake. By the same mechanism, we all have a pre-verbal memory that alarms us that a loss of love is potentially lethal.

We may balk at the way some scientists will extend the concept of *joy* to rats, we may doubt if *grief* in elephants is as intense or prolonged as human grief, and we may object that *empathy* in mice does not convey the same meaning as the empathy that funds our humanitarian institutions. Scientists use these words because the physiological manifestations are similar in all mammals. Emotions in animals serve the same purpose as emotions in humans: they bond animals with one another and regulate behaviors relative to sexuality, parenting, food distribution, cooperation, competition, aggression and escape. Even the so called "spindle cells," which were long thought to exist only in humans or in great apes, have been discovered to be present in other mammals. These cells and their location in the brain are responsible for social organization, empathy, and intuition about the feelings of others. We are moved by accounts of elephants who suffer from depression because they are separated from their companion; it confirms that a loss of friendship can cause serious symptoms. Indeed elephants, dogs, horses, bears, dolphins... do show symptoms of all sorts of psychosomatic disturbance: depression, post-traumatic stress disorder, and even character disorders which can make them incompetent parents[16] and lousy friends. This kind of animal research is very convincing: not only do elephants grieve, but, because they live so long, they develop a magnificent limbic capacity from which disenfranchised humans could learn a thing or two! For example, every member of their group can locate all the others at any given moment and elephants seem to instinctively know who needs help, where, and how to comfort each other. They also spend a huge amount of their time, up to one third of their waking hours, fondling and caressing each other with their trunks, a soothing and bonding activity. We humans might consider imitating elephants, instead of medicating the consequences of our busyness and loneliness.[17]

Since our limbic/emotional brain is responsible for the survival mechanisms we share with mammals, it explains how a person who just lost his most important relationship emits signals of distress similar to any other abandoned mammal. Your wimps and meows, howling and growling might take the form of repeated phone calls, obsessive emailing, begging for the return of love, yet, whatever the form in which you express your distress, your state of alarm is chemically identical to that of the abandoned pup or baby.[18] The kitten that can't access the tit, the child who can't find the mother in the mall, and the adult who is separated from the habitual loving partner suffer the exact same limbic distress. Consider yourself like a pup who has been kicked out in the cold winter night and is crying at the door.

Expressions of emotional distress occur only in species that have developed a limbic brain, which is to say only when a cry for help has a chance of receiving an answer in the form of rescue. The salmon caught in the net doesn't send a signal of distress to its mommy, because the baby salmon has no limbic brain, nor does the mommy salmon; it has no capacity to experience pain or panic. Same for the crocodile: it looks at its offspring being squashed by a bulldozer without any fuss at all! Crocodile's tears are indeed not emotional tears while a kitten's meow is a different matter; the cat has a limbic brain and the kitten does express a distress to which the mother will respond. With human adults experiencing separation anxiety, not only is the activity of the brain similar to that of mammals in distress, the *sequence* of reactions is also the same. An abandoned pup, as well as the human baby, first begins to protest loudly, which, in the animal world, is an auditory signal for the rescuing parent to locate the lost pup.

Bowlby's classical studies on loss and attachment were the first to incorporate observations from the animal world into theories of psychoanalysis. Although Bowlby's attachment theory was initially rejected by the establishment of Freudian orthodoxy, his empirical observations became known for their accuracy and are now confirmed by neuroscience. For example, what Bowlby called the initial "protest phase" shows an increase in heart rate and body temperature, and a surge in the levels of the stress hormones (catecholamine and cortisol). The effect of catecholamine is similar to that of adrenaline: it raises alertness, as we see in the hypervigilance of a child afraid that dad may be drunk again and hit him at any minute. It is the same anxious hypervigilance that makes us nervous and jumpy when we feel somebody is trying to seduce our partner. This state of hypervigilance is also what makes us see the partner who recently abandoned us, in every car that vaguely resembles the partner's car. That first phase of protest cannot last very long before somatic deterioration starts to happen. When rescue does not come, the little mammal slowly loses the strength to howl; Bowlby called that phase *despair*. It is followed by a state of neurological sluggishness that Bowlby described as a *failure to thrive*, or *miasma*. The word *miasma* is an interesting one; in ancient Greece it meant a form of *pollution* of the body/ soul connection[19]. Bowlby's concept of *miasma* defines a physiological state where the body just gives up trying to get love. Loss of love and depression are such similar states that scientists who study the chemistry of depression use separation from the animal mother to produce depressed experimental rats.[20] Neuroscientists could as well study your brain, if they could access it as you cry into your pillows, because lovesickness is one such state of *miasma*.

As Bowlby observed, the longer abandonment and miasma persist, the more the immune system weakens. As the emotional stress moves from acute to chronic, the learning centers deteriorate, the young mammal (including babies) eventually refuses nourishment, and soon dies. We now know the mechanisms by which the brain of an unloved child, to whom no one speaks and with whom no one plays, deteriorates so completely that the capacity to develop language can be lost forever. We all know that children need love, songs, play, interactions, challenges they can solve, caresses, smiles, tickling, surprises, joy...not only because it is the moral thing to do with our little ones, but because if they don't get it, their limbic brain stops developing. Scientists have studied the effect of love deprivation on the brains of orphaned children for almost a century and Bowlby's original 'attachment theory' has branched out in the fields of neuropsychology, evolutionary psychology and ethological theory. Attachment theories now include the study of trauma and attachment patterns in adults [21] and demonstrate how loss of love in adult life can turn into a major trauma. Yet, with all this convincing research, it seems that our culture ignores the fact that isolated adults suffering from heartbreak need more than a week off from work *to get over it* and *move on.*

You must take into consideration that your grief can make you less capable than a trained rat in its familiar maze! *All* individuals experiencing the loss of the most important love relationship report cognitive impairments: "I can't do my work, I'll read a whole page of a report, and I barely understand what the sentences mean...I can't concentrate, I keep making stupid mistakes, I can't think straight, I function at such a low level I dread going to work..." Habitual neural circuits are deranged and this neuronal disorder translates as neuronal sluggishness. If it lasts, there is synaptic degeneration. Love is the strongest life-sustaining factor; to see the person who provides it suddenly departing or dying is terrifying and somatically dangerous. Heartbreak is a trauma; as if it wasn't enough to suffer it in the present, it is also inevitably amplified by past traumas[22]. As you are a mammal, you can't avoid the instinctual limbic urge to protest, howl, cry, beg, although it takes a somewhat different form. Love songs are overwhelmingly calls of distress and protest, to which the artist adds poetry and music. Love songs express, in one form or another, the archetypal basic plea: "Don't be cruel to a heart that's true"[23] and they repeat it over and over. The artistic variations are endless, yet the theme is timeless and universal: without the partner, the world is a desolate place, a desert.

Young mammals go from the initial phase of protest to the final stage of miasma in a consistent order. In human adults, the movement from the protest phase (the "Don't be cruel" plea) to the stage of despairing depression and miasma (the gamut of feelings expressed in the blues...) can be interwoven, going back and forth between protest and depression, depression and miasma, miasma and angry protest, alternating the crying and the begging with depression in a darkened bedroom or jumpiness at the workplace. What is to be done with such misery?

Some environments, some friends are such that they *console* and *reassure*: two ordinary words that mean the same as what neuroscientists mean by "limbic regulation" or "affect regulation." Reassuring and creating safety is also what a therapist does when faced with a patient in acute psychological distress. Some therapists, some friends, some milieus are more consoling than others.[24] One finds the opposite of consolation and reassurance in milieus where productivity and competition are pushed to a level that provokes limbic distress. It does help to find consolation and support in a group, yet, as we shall see in the next chapter where I discuss the limitations of grief counseling, it is not enough if all that you do is to tell you story over and over again, until all your friends and family start taking their distance from such a sad character as yourself. For sure, if you join a group, visit family, go on a cruise, eat out, go to the cinema, cook for friends, cook with friends, take tango lessons, join a choir, do volunteer work, start therapy... the presence of other has the power to reassure the lost, frightened, abandoned, primitive little person in you. In fact, anything that activates the pleasure principle (laughter, a massage, a good meal...even masturbation[25]) can be considered "limbic regulation" and is helpful, yet not the whole story.

That lost pup that resides in your limbic brain needs not only your compassion but also some reassurance that pleasure is still possible. Just like a crying child can be consoled by a hug and an ice cream cone, it is important to find what works for your adult self. A study on friendship among women revealed an interesting way of coping with stress at the workplace: bonding and befriending. Drs. Klein and Taylor at UCLA[26] discovered that friendship releases oxytocin—the hormone of bonding between mother and baby. This substance is also produced by men, but not when testosterone dominates their reaction. This study confirms many previous studies that demonstrated how social ties reduce our risk of disease by lowering blood pressure, heart rate, and cholesterol.[27] Similarly, a good massage, an acupuncture treatment, a session of meditation may also produce somatic benefits by lowering the stress response.

When Jung was formulating his theory of individuation, he was influenced by the Indian yogic system of lower and higher chakras. Living from one's lower two chakras exemplifies the concept of living from one's animal nature. The process of individuation is certainly not a denial of the lower instincts, but the highest possible development of the higher chakras, which qualify us as humans and is the key to the liberation of the heart.

It is time to introduce the last actor in the drama of heartbreak, the one who can individuate, the human capable of wisdom.

3) The wise, mindful human (neocortex)
The fact that children make and need attachment

objects has been used in much psychoanalytic theory as a guide, or blueprint, for adult sexual relations. But this model brings with it the idea that the value or quality of a relationship is measured by its duration and fidelity. 'Good' relationships become those in which people can tolerate a lot of frustration, as children, indeed, have to do [...]. In psychoanalytic stories it is as though the adult is always succumbing to the child within. But it is one of the advantages of growing up that one can extend the repertoire of possible relationships.

Adam Philips [28]

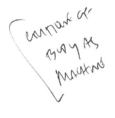

Emotional life can be influenced, but it cannot be commanded. Our society's love affair with mechanical devices that respond at a button-touch ill prepares us to deal with the unruly organic mind that dwells within. Anything that does not comply must be broken or poorly designed, people now suppose, including their hearts.

(Lewis, Amini, Lannon.)[29]

We cannot detach at will from the rejecting or deceased partner because we cannot control the brain, yet, we may relate to the emotions with some measure of distance (again: this is called *affect regulation*[30]). The dominant cultural myth for many generations has made us think of our bodies as machines that should run without defect until the very end, so that when it breaks down, we feel like a wreaked car. The approach of the wise human is different: it is not to try to control the brain (we can't), not to try to fix the mechanic (we are not machines), but rather to *relate* to the crocodile and the pup. In this relating, adaptation will happen.[31] Healing from grief is not a fixing of a defective machine because it is more like an *education*, with the same depth of transformation. The neocortical development that qualifies us as humans gave us the use of language, the ability to write, the capacity for logical and formal operational thinking. It also gave us the abilities that are responsible for the development of the arts and the humanities because we humans need to symbolize, metaphorize and invent stories. We imagine ahead, we daydream, we fantasize; and it is only after the deployment of imagination that we are motivated to use rational means to make our dreams come true. You'll need to update absolutely all those connections: the symbolic and the factual, the right emotional hemisphere as well as the left rational hemisphere.

Mammals do have a cerebral cortex, variable in size; for example, the cortex of a rabbit is pitifully small compared to that of a dog, which is why no magician was ever able to teach a rabbit to curtsy as it comes out of the hat. The human cortex is proportionally twice as big as that of any other mammal, and with abilities that are unique. As our neocortical neural structure evolved, we developed not only the capacity for sophisticated language, art, science, music, but also a capacity to love at the deep level that we do. Humans yearn for the fullest possible experience of love, which can exist only at the highest level of our evolution.

Puppy love and the symbiotic attachment of mother and child are foundational, beautiful and necessary, and certainly the bond with our pet animal can be gratifying and cozy, but it is not the full expression of the human capacity to love, nor is the disturbance of the limbic regulation the full expression of the catastrophe of human heartbreak.

The challenge involved in *relating* with the specifically human part of our brain, lies in the fact that the brain development that gives us the capacity to observe empirically, to theorize, to invent and experiment does not protect us against false demonstrations, destructive beliefs, a language that lies, logical mistakes, uninformed theories and rationalizations that have little to do with rationality. In other words, although we do have the capacity to be wise and rational, we are not necessarily up to the task, nor do we, at times, wish to be. Heartbreak, along with fear and rage, are ultimate demonstrations of the fact that our rational brain, like our ego, is not always the captain of our ship. The neocortical capacities are the seat of the greatest leaps in the evolution of human culture; yet, when we are heartbroken, our whole brain engages in a chaotic neuronal dance which brings back on stage the other two actors, the crocodile and the pup. Together, all three actors engage in reckless strategies in a desperate effort to control the supply of love. This is why we have a rational code of law, which, fortunately, is there to limit our more primitive impulses. It is our rational capacity that reminds us: "If I break into the partner's apartment, against the judge's restriction order,

I'll go to prison, so I won't." Willpower, self-control, good manners, as well as the code of law, help most of us avoid prison, which is not to say that we are free of crocodile impulses and puppy distress.

Getting an education is a simple but not a simplistic process: you go to a school, you listen, read, discuss, relate, write, think, talk, tackle difficult problems, and you do it for as long as it takes for your brain to be trained. Being indoctrinated into a destructive cult follows the same process: you stay with the ideas and the people for long enough for your brain to be modified. What makes the difference between an education that frees you and an education that enslaves you are the ideas, the persons, the values, the challenges that are offered by the milieu one is joining to get that education. The education offered in a cultish milieu is based on one great simplistic illusion: follow a bible of some sort, or follow an authority figure (guru, priest, pope, chief), do like him, think like him, do this, do that, don't do this, don't do that, don't think for yourself, obey… and you'll be saved. Not even in my very own tribe of Jungians and archetypal psychologists are we immune to the danger of trying to imitate someone else's process of individuation.[32] The heartbroken person is especially at risk of replacing the love addiction to the lost partner with an addiction to an authority figure, because one wants so much to *believe* in some superior power that can offer rescue. By contrast, the kind of education that you need is one that frees your mind and heart, augments your autonomy and your critical sense, as opposed to some puffy theory like *The Secret*[33]. Simplicity is beautiful; simplification is dangerous. Positive thinking is crucial, but as Ehrenreich's (2009) recent research has shown, the relentless promotion of positive thinking can have terrible side effects. The worst example I can give of a that of a young woman whose goal was to graduate from college and she was led to believe that she would pass the exam if she slept with the book under her pillow and *visualized* herself with the cap an gown of a graduate. She believed in this magic instead of studying the subject matter, and failed. Simplistic approaches not only fail when a real obstacle presents itself, they also add to the collective burden of ignorance by confusing science with magical thinking, psychology with hocus-pocus tricks.

The plasticity of the brain is like an appetite for learning: if you feed it junk, it produces junk knowledge. As your goal is freedom from grief, you need to learn as much as you can about the psychology of the crocodile, the psychology of the pup, to avoid replacing one form of addiction with another.

What I mean by *getting an education* is not to get a diploma, but rather to open up to the deeper aspects of learning, ones that touch both the heart and the intellect and activate neurogenesis. One could as well use a psycho-spiritual term: *being initiated*, because both the notions of *education* and that of *initiation* imply an intense intellectual adventure, combined with an intense emotional engagement. For example getting your driving license when you come of age is a huge initiation: one has to *learn* the skills of driving a car, and once you learn how to drive a car, you never forget it, it is part of your procedural memories inscribed in the brain. But getting your first driver's license is also an emotional, transitional moment, because, in our culture, the capacity and the legal right to drive a car is one of the most potent symbol of the coming of age. Education and initiation are experiences that define a *before* and an *after,* which is another way of saying that the synaptic connections are changed in a permanent way. The process can be scary because it pushes us to the next level of our evolution. Getting an education, being initiated, is like that: scary, necessary, and fantastically interesting, as the next chapter will try to demonstrate.

CHAPTER 3

RECOVERING

*A good study for equilibrating our suffering
has yet to be written. It is surprising, since
humanity has been suffering for quite a time.
For moral suffering, we have a bit more know-
how, although there are still many a fool who,
when faced with misfortune, will search for
the counterweight, not of another misfortune,
but of happiness!*

Henri Michaux. [34]

Brain training

The principles of education have been the same since
humans began educating their young, they are *simple*, as
opposed to simplistic. Getting an education is simple, but
it takes time and devotion, and it is not focused exclusively
on the positive, the angelic, the miraculous, the artificial
boosting of self-esteem. To drive a car, one has to develop
a very clear image of how this machine can kill you, kill
others, and send you to prison, because a car is one of the
most dangerous object in our cultural environment. It is also

an object that can augment one's freedom, if you learn to use it properly. Learning to drive is simple, yet there is a learning curve about it, as well as an emotional and even moral dimension to it.

Every psychologist will agree that it is important to have a positive outlook on life, and a psychotherapist's task is to use every possible means to enhance the placebo response (imagining a positive outcome) and decrease the nocebo effect (fantasies of gloom and doom that act as self-fulfilling prophecies).[35] Hypnotic techniques can enhance the powerful placebo effect by replacing negative suggestions with positive ones. Anything that augments the placebo effect and decrease the nocebo effect has its function in healing.[36] Both the nocebo and the placebo effects are very real, yet one cannot have transformation if one ignores the negative and the neurotic –what Jungians call the shadow. Ignoring the shadow is no way to awaken that *wise human* who can get you through grief. Psychologists and neuroscientists agree on the basic principle of all psychotherapies: unconscious conflicts translate into physical symptoms, repeated failures, and broken relationships. If you refuse to look at your bag of neurosis, your body will carry the conflict. A heartbreak brings our unconscious conflicts to the surface; it is as if we had in the brain a software that translated psychological distress into physical discomfort, to bring our attention to a situation that needs to change. The less conscious we are, the more we rely on the alarm system that *has* to make our body sick to get our attention. *The body always carries what the psyche does not want to see!* One aspect of the work of psychotherapy is to re-translate back the physical symptom into its original emotional source, to deal with the conflict at the level at which it is happening, in order to spare the body. When the problem has a strictly medical cause, a strictly medical solution will fix it; but when for example, we are *worried sick*, it is safer and wiser to start with the worry, not the sickness, although Big Pharma wants us to believe the opposite. This retranslation of the physical into the psychological is the way of the *wise human* in you. Jung called it *individuation* and wrote about it as the most interesting adventure of human life.

Start the process of neurogenesis

People break up for the same reasons they get together– a mix of healthy motives and neurotic complexes. No one escapes a measure of neurosis around love, because we all have a need for love which conflicts with our need for freedom. Because of that conflict, our need for love (an instinctual one) is necessarily mixed with *fear*. That fear is felt as a tension between opposites: the fear of losing love and the fear of loving, because love may restrict the freedom necessary to discover one's own identity. It is the neurotic contamination of love with fear that breaks the heart, never love itself. A break-up becomes a breakthrough when it forces the letting go of some of the neurotic aspects of love as addiction. The telluric intensity of heartbreak can actually cut through a layer of our complexes and addictions like fire destroys decay, because our heart is as wide-open in grief as it was to love's bliss. If you can tolerate staying with the pain and keep your heart open, the pain will force your brain to re-organize its synaptic connections to adapt to the new situation.

Our brain learns by defeat as much as by victory, by pain as much as by joy, by positive as well as negative conditioning; it reacts as powerfully to the placebo effect (positive suggestion) as to the nocebo effect (negative suggestion). The brain is eager to learn but does so only when faced with either an intense pleasure or a pressing problem. It is economical to ignore what seems to work but it is dangerous to ignore what hurts. The abandonment by your partner is now sending an urgent call to your brain: do something, quick! At first, your brain reacts like that of a drug addict suddenly deprived of his/her drug, which explains why the behavior of the love-crazy is similar to that of the addict desperately searching for a fix. In your case, the "fix" is the abandoner. Calling every ten minutes to leave messages on the answering machine, ("where are you, why don't you come back, who are you with, I can't live without you, don't leave me"…), a deluge of emails, a long wait in one's car to see him/her appear, crying and begging, trying every possible strategy to get the other to come back are all typical behaviors of the phase were the addiction emerges. Hooked on hope, your brain is in a panic mode. When asked "what exactly is this panic, what are you afraid of, really?," the answer is always extravagant, something like "without him/her, my life is over, worthless, boring, I can't live without him/her." This obsessive impulsivity is typical of the first phase of a heartbreak. It is no surprise that failures of love are at the core of most depressive, suicidal states and often lead to drug or alcohol addiction. You should know that your brain does not differentiate between the lack of love, the lack of food, or the lack of sleep. A threat is a threat. At this very crucial point, you have to make a choice: either you stay in that passive, panicky and victimizing mode, which leads to stagnation, or manipulative strategies and revenge, or humiliation and a closed heart, or you start considering the options.

The limitations of grief counseling

The United States invented a profession called "grief counselor". It is so popular that there are now many areas of specialization, and one can even get an online certification on Pet Loss Grief Counseling. There are grief counselors in hospices, hospitals, schools, in local community groups, online, and on site. They intervene when a collective trauma occurs and they offer a form of "companioning" that has its merits. Grief therapy can calm the limbic panic which inevitably occurs whenever there is a major disruption of one's physical or emotional environment. The security of a group is just what the mammalian brain needs to calm down. A support group is, to the human individual, what the wolf pack is to the wolf pup. Grief therapy can prevent panic, and often has a calming effect that is more powerful than most medication.

Yet, it has its limitations. One of the basic tenet of such an approach is that grief happens in stages – not the stages identified by Bowlby's careful study of animal behavior– but rather the stages theorized by Elizabeth Kübler-Ross[37] in the seventies: anger, bargaining, depression, acceptance. As Konigsberg (2011) recently pointed out, Kübler-Ross's theory was not the result of careful empirical observations –unlike Bowlby's rigorous empirical study of animal behavior– but only a hypothesis formulated after a few interviews with dying patients. Her hypothesis that grief happens in stages, according to Konigsberg, was never put to the test.[38] Many of my own students, who counsel the heartbroken and the bereaved, are surprised when they learn that Kübler-Ross was not referring to mourning the loss of a loved one, but rather the acceptance of one's imminent death. And finally, their certitude about the healing effects of "telling one's story" is shaken when they discover that it depends on *how* one is telling the story. For example, a study by Bonnano (2007)[39] suggests that there might be more benefits in a form of "repressive coping", a notion that seems to me quite close to what used to be called good manners and self-restraint. As my grandmother used to say: "if you are going to cry in the soup, you better stay in your bedroom." Of course, she was right, because sadness is not attractive, and telling your sad story to everyone who will hear it eventually isolates you. A grief counselor might not object to your obsessive re-telling, because he/she gets paid for listening, but friends and family will resent your whining.

Neuroscience does confirm that the narrative function is an important part of our cognitive abilities, yet not every form of narrative will have a healing effect. If you keep repeating the story of *who* did *what*, to *whom*, *how*, it may be useful in the beginning, yet if it goes on too long, it becomes counter-productive. The kind of story telling that does *not* work looks like a list of grievances and facts: "she took the kids…he left me with no money… she lied to me… he cheated for years before I found out… she wiped our accounts… he lied about his assets… she turned the kids against me … he did not give me any warning and just left a letter… she changed her phone number and put a new lock on her door… blah, blah, blah… on and on with the facts and the complaining. It keeps you focused on your pain, on your grievances, because it keeps you stuck in the limbic aspect of your disappointment: the moaning, complaining, whining, of the lost pup. Telling the facts over and over again, as a child tells the story to mommy, can be consoling, it may even be necessary, but only up to a point. The brain won't oblige to reconfigure itself until you move up in the ladder of evolution. Grief counseling can console and calm the frightened pup in our limbic brain, it can offer company when loneliness is too much to bear, and it prevents a dangerous form of isolation. Yet, it is not enough and you must now learn to use the full repertoire of symbolic expression; in others words, you need to engage the part of the brain that is specifically human. Instead of repeating *who did what to whom*, you must find the symbols and metaphors that will situate you.

Carl Jung is probably the psychologist who best explained how attention to the *emerging symbols* can augment consciousness. You have to understand that the resolution of your heartbreak is *not* limited to the re-establishment of a limbic sense of secure attachment; it is much more than that. Jung called it the process of individuation, where the pain of heartbreak brings about a new conscious standpoint, one that transcends the previous opposition between love and hate, security and freedom. The process of individuation is like a quest for wisdom, a life-long fascinating adventure, a process of withdrawal of more and more projections, a continuous recognition of more contradictory impulses within oneself, leading to ever-increasing levels of consciousness. Paying attention to the symbols that resonate in our psyche is the key to the process of individuation. Many approaches now concur with Jung's basic intuition of the power of symbols and metaphors to impact emotions.

Finding the emerging symbols

It would help us to put our troubles "outside" us and make them function as if they were images."

Gaston Bachelard[40]

*If one is to learn theology on oneself, one
expects to discover religion's images to be
precise metaphoric expressions of that which
one thinks and feels: thrown into a world
where things need naming; expulsed from
Edenic sense; towering Babel; flooding in life;
bondage; walking dry through the midst of
seas; wandering in wildernesses; drawn to gold
idols; wanting a king like the others; exiled; on
a ash heap; whirlwind; something sacred being
born out of a virginal place in the self; nailed;
betrayed; miraculously going on; waiting for
the spirit to come; apocalypse now; my God,
why hast thou forsaken me. "*

David Miller[41]

Telling the facts is not enough, but finding the images
and metaphors for your situation will force an opening of
your imagination, which, in itself, pushes you beyond the
whining pup.

The week after his shock at Laura's lack of compassion
for his distress, William began writing down his feelings.
He could not stop feeling cold and he was often shivering
and was wondering what was going on. The act of writing
opened his imagination, to reveal a vast choice of metaphors
to symbolize his emotional state. He wrote that he was *a
turtle dying within its shell.* Eureka! This metaphor gave
him a most valuable information because he immediately
understood the psychosomatic damage happening in his
body (the turtle is dying) and the urgency for him to reach
out of his turtle shelf. Out of his *turtled* self!

I AM A TURTLE DYING IN ITS SHELL

Last night, having some regrets at the way she treated me when I delivered her mail, Laura called me and suggested that we should have dinner together. Our separation was never quite final and although I have good days, where I can feel that my obsession with Laura is abating, there is still a part of me that remains hooked on hope. I was getting excited at the idea that she might tell me that having Jack move in with her was not such a success... hope, hope, my enemy.

So, after work, I went to the supermarket to get the ingredients to cook a gourmet dinner. I opened an exceptionally fine bottle of Burgundy, flowers on the table, music... everything was ready at six, but she arrived forty minutes late, distracted, dressed in jeans and a t-shirt, as if she had come from the gym. She gulped in exactly ten minutes the gourmet dinner that had taken me an hour to prepare, swallowing without tasting. Her eyes avoided mine, no relaxing into the experience of eating, no melting in each other's presence, as a good meal used to do for us. I felt she had come not because she really wanted to evaluate how things are between us, but because she felt guilty: she likes to think of herself as a compassionate being, a pacifist, a loving soul. Laura adopts lost dogs and cats, feeds birds, plants trees; she participates in programs to heal the ocean, heal the forest, preserve wild horses, preserve the rain forest and preserve the ozone layer. She will not boil a live lobster and does not approve of foie gras and she won't travel to China because they eat dogs and cats. She is a do-gooder and absolutely cannot face the fact that she not only betrayed me, but lied to me and lacked compassion when I was in shock at her door. Do-gooders are the most dangerous partners: they torture you while remaining innocent.

We had barely finished dinner when she got up to start the dishes (the Good Girl again). When done, the good girl thanked me for the delicious dinner and then stabbed me with the kind of lies good girls will do when they are unconscious of their dark sides: "excuse me darling, I have an avalanche of emails to answer tonight. This was lovely, I loved seeing you, and it was important for me to re-establish our friendship. You know how much I love you and I would not want to hurt you. We don't know what the future of our relationship might hold. Let's remain friends. Now, I must get home early." I knew without a doubt that she was going to spend the rest of the weekend with Jack. Laura's quick peck on my cheek, at the doorstep, felt like a slap in the face, a blow disguised as a kiss, her form of emotional lie. She left, probably feeling she was still a compassionate person, because she had visited me tonight. Stupid me!

As soon as she left, I began having heart palpitations. I finally realized how utterly defeated I was; abandoned, rejected, unloved and unchosen, lied to, manipulated, and used, lonely and vulnerable. I went to bed early and at 2:00 a.m., I woke up thinking I was having a heart attack. I ended up at the hospital emergency, only to be told I was having "stress cardiomyopathy." I came back heavily sedated, to a cold nest.

I am a turtle dying in its shell.

The symbolic and the medical have long been presented by the medical establishment as opposite point of views, a terrible mistake that the recent understanding of the psyche/soma connection is correcting. A heartbreak happens in the brain, in the heart, and in the imagination. Like love, heartbreak is a symbolic, biological, psychological, spiritual event and nothing about it can be limited to an either/or simplistic interpretations. To recover from heartbreak, one needs *both* an adequate symbolization *and* adequate medical attention. William's visit to the hospital and the diagnosis he was given were essential; yet, this is not what convinced him of the urgency for more detachment. What really got his attention was the symbol of the turtle dying in its shell. This image, this embodied metaphor got right through the heart of the problem: a turtle dying in its shell is a clear enough image. Symbols and metaphors are the most powerful avenues of communication between the conscious and unconscious realms.

Jerome Bruner was a pioneer in using the language of cognitive psychology to state what Jung and others, in the humanities and the arts have long known. Reading Bruner today feels as if cognitive psychologists want everybody to believe that they discovered, all by themselves, the power of metaphors, myths and symbols. A little humility would be nice from Bruner and his followers, who seem to lack a basic education in the humanities. They appear unaware that they reframe basic ideas that philosophers, psychoanalysts and literary geniuses have long expressed. Bruner's influence came to dominate cognitive psychology[42] and his book *The Process of Education*, inspired the US Head Start project. In *Acts of Meaning*[43] Bruner educated the behavioral-cognitive psychologists about the meaning-making capacity of formulating a narrative. He convinced those who may have never read a novel in their life, or those who don't even know what a metaphor is, that a narrative not only *organizes* experience, it also *constructs reality*. If you have an education in the arts and the humanities, you already understand that. What Bruner calls the *agentive self,* is what in literature is called, simply, the protagonist, or hero. Bruner repeatedly insisted on the power of metaphor, metonymy, synecdoche, implicature and all the literary tricks that give us the possibility to speak figuratively instead of literally. In Bruner's terms, when William found his metaphor of the turtle dying in its shell, he was *organizing and framing his experience,* an activity which in turn influences his *personal affect regulation* (behavioral-cognitive jargon for "feelings").

The ancient Greeks had a more concise and elegant word to mean the *organizing and framing of one's experience*: "poiesis," a term too often translated as meaning the writing of a poem in verse. Its original meaning is much more interesting: a poeisis is the shaping of something into a coherent *form,* like when you take wood planks and make them in the form of a table with four legs. A *form* is needed to create an object, and it is needed to communicate an emotion. Shaping your life's drama into a series of evolving metaphors, and into stories is a *poiesis.* A beautiful story is not one where you embellish the facts and add a happy ending, but rather one that communicates the emotional truth with precision and depth. To use the words of Harold Bloom, [44] "our despair requires consolation, and the medicine of a profound narration."

We may not all have the literary genius of a Goethe, who, being rejected by Charlotte Buff, took care of his suicidal depression by writing *The Sorrows of Young Werther.* His was an economical solution: instead of killing himself in despair, Goethe has the young Werther commit suicide. As James Hillman so eloquently argues, there is no need to literalize a physical suicide when a symbolic one will do.[45] Stendhal used that same medicine of a *profound narration* when, out of his despair at not being able to marry into nobility, he wrote the1822's classic *On Love*. Stendhal's obsession with Countess Dembowska led him to formulate the concept of *crystallization* which he defines as "that operation of the mind which turns whatever presents, itself into a discovery of new perfections in the object of love," a concept identical to what psychologists today call the *idealization of the love object*. Stendhal believed that being too isolated, too lonely, as he was at the time, was the breeding ground for *crystallization*. Analyzing the various stages of his love obsession, he rightly observed that in love, everything is a sign, ("tout est signe en amour")– which, by the way, is true not only with love obsession, like Stendhal's obsession with the Countess, but also in states of jealousy and paranoia. Becoming an expert on his own love madness did not spare him the dark emotions, but *formulating* them was the key to turn his heartbreak into a breakthrough.

With or without a literary talent, there is something in the neurological makeup of our left hemisphere that seeks not only an *explanation* for why an event occurs but also an image and a *story* about it. Michael Gazzaniga, who, along with Joseph LeDoux, is credited with launching the field of *cognitive neuroscience* in the early 1980, calls that need for a narrative the *interpreter mechanism* of the brain. He describes it as the "creative, narrative talent of the left hemisphere"[46], as opposed to *literalist attitude* of the right hemisphere. Although both hemispheres can be viewed as conscious, the left brain's consciousness is the one who not only wants to create a narrative of the heartbreak, but can be truly satisfied with the suicide of a fictional character. This need for a narration is precisely what depth psychologists have been writing about, helping patient formulate their metaphors and stories. William is no Stendhal or Goethe, yet the image of a turtle dying in its shell was a precise symbolization of his impending psychic death. Writing about this turtle in his notebook worked just like writing the suicide of *Young Werther*. It situated him: "you are psychically dying, will you do something about this?"

Even in severely abusive situations, such as the next vignette about Debbie's relationship to Bob, the metaphorizing of the abuse can help the person see how the abuse can feel so *natural*. Debbie, at the first therapy session, described her lover as an abuser and herself as the victim! Therapy helped her see that theirs was a matching neurosis that bound them together. Although on a conscious level she saw Bob as an abuser, on an unconscious level she believed that she was born to be used ("I'm trash") while Bob was entitled to be served ("He's royalty"). Royalty, if one looks at human history, used to be thought of as a divine right, the result of God's will. Debbie could not think otherwise, because Bob's abuse felt so natural to her.

I'M TRASH AND HE'S ROYALTY

For the last five years, Bob has not paid his share of the rent, nor of the food, nor of any other expenses because he has been working only part time and paying off debts. I am older than he by 15 years, earn a lot more than he does, I have a nest egg in the bank, and I could afford giving him free room and board. I believed it would be a temporary situation, maybe a few months. After five years of that regimen, his student loan was finally paid off, and he began actively searching for a job. Finally, last month, he got a full time job. Instead of offering to contribute to our common expenses, he bought himself a thirty foot sail boat, the cost of which made it impossible to start paying me rent. He said he absolutely needed a big «ego-booster,» something to rescue him from a sense of worthlessness and depression after the five years of unemployment!

I could not brush off my disappointment and I insisted on his financial participation, but that is not what happened. He decided that it would be a good thing for our relationship if he had his «own space,» which meant living on his sailing boat. A little voice in me whispered: he has been using you all along! I am an obese woman, and Bob has ways of making me feel like trash because of my weight. I too feel like trash. That is why I have been willing to be his sugar mommy and pay for everything all this time. Now that he has the means to afford his own space he wants freedom from mommy. I may be a big woman, but I won't be a sugar mommy anymore, I want a man, not a boy. I am working on restoring a sense of respect for myself, body and soul. My heartbreak over Bob is a good thing: it is a wake up call.

Complementary neurosis are hard to pin-point, and often finding the right metaphor for the situation helps bring about a breakup which is a healthy response from a psyche that wants to break free. It was the case for Debbie.

DEBBIE'S COMPLACENCY

Regardless of the actual reason for his rudeness, Bob's basic implicit message to me was this: «whatever you do, I'll never let you make me happy. What you feel is of no interest to me. Shut-up so I can talk. Move over, so I can have center stage. Tell me if you plan on crying, so I can bolt. Take care of everything, but don't take any initiative. You're really my servant, but I don't want you to know this. More than anything else, don't you become aware of the fact that I do not love you. After all, you are still useful to me. I plan to keep you around.» I have taken Bob's abuse for so long, my will is broken, my passion for life is quenched. I am a zombie.

Debbie's brain developed in a family where abuse and harsh manners was the *natural* state of affairs but she could not see that. A rejected or abused child remains with the abusive family because freedom is not yet a viable option; survival first, quality of life... later. A teenager indoctrinated to become a suicide bomber is not really free to refuse martyrdom; an abused child, a wife in an fundamentalist patriarchal culture; an adolescent raised in a war zone, in a drug culture, educated in a school where violence is tolerated... all remain blind to the abuse because it always was there; it has become the standard. Debbie stayed with Bob because she looked at him with a child's eyes, still living by the values that were prevalent in her abusive family. She found them painful but *natural*, just like the majority of women in fiercely sexist milieus find it absolutely *natural* to be deprived of the rights given to men. These women will resist feminist ideas. For Debbie, the influence of a new set of values, through her participation in the writing group at the city college, had on her the effect of a revolutionary ferment. The workshop on memoir writing was hosted by a retired professor of literature, at the local community college. With the help from the group and from reading the books[47], Debbie realized what it meant to be a *zombie*. The image was a shock. The shock was fertile ground for her late blooming.

She discovered that although a child cannot face the terror of abandonment, an adult can. It took the cultural influence of the group, *and* its emotional support, to convince her that she was strong enough to refuse Bob's abuse; that she could live from a different set of values. In the writing exercises with the memoir group, she expressed how, as a child, she waited to receive the visit of her father, who never came. The group taking interest in Debbie's writing gave her a taste of what parental attention can feel like, in other words, the group was a good parent. She wrote how, all her life, she waited for some form of expression of affection from her mother, whom she served with devotion, without receiving as much as a thank you. The support of the other women in the group was her first taste of motherly acceptance. She was being *re-parented* as psychologists say. She eventually saw how her prison was self-imposed and how her need to be coupled was contrary to love. The workshop leader gave them only one guideline, one that is basic in therapy: do not ask "why" but rather "how": "*how* do I restrict my freedom of movement, *how* do I live like a zombie, *how* to I let Bob abuse me?

Debbie came to see the connection between her fear of freedom and her shallow breathing. She wrote: "there is plenty of oxygen (freedom) out there, but I am unable to take much in; my breathing is the shallowest when I am around Bob." Her writing and re-writing of her story, the reading of it to the other participants, helped her move out of her addiction to a destructive relationship. The text Debbie wrote about her divorce had the tone of liberation and celebration. She wrote: "my divorce papers are like the *emancipation papers* slaves were given when freed by the master." A metaphor needs to change when the situation evolves. To avoid psychic rigidity, we must keep on refreshing our album of images. Debbie's metaphor evolved and instead of *emancipation papers*, her divorce became her *Declaration of Independence*. She wrote: "I self-govern! I have stopped imagining that freedom was *given* to me by a master. I prefer to imagine that I declared my war of Independence and won. It is more active than waiting for a master to hand you freedom." The move from her first metaphor to the second one beautifully expresses the progression of her psychological strength.

We resort to metaphor each time we need to explain something unfamiliar or mysterious by comparing it to something familiar or simple. If you say "heartbreak is an emotional tsunami," you are using the well-known meteorological phenomenon to explain the less known emotional reality of heartbreak. To communicate with others, scientists cannot avoid using metaphors, although they call it "a mapping from the source domain to the target domain."[48] Any given metaphor, in any field, is useful as long it helps the thinking; it becomes problematic when it prevents new thinking. For example, the choice of a metaphor for the phenomenon of the "folding" of proteins is an interesting story. In their efforts to understand how proteins seem to "fold," biochemists had to ask themselves if proteins fold like folding chairs and folding bicycles, along rigid pre-defined lines, or do they fold like a napkin or a sheet of paper, wherever pressure is applied? Or could it be that *folding* is the wrong image and that it would be more accurate to talk about a *rolling* of the protein, like one rolls a scroll, or like a *coiling* rope? Each of these nuances can be responsible either for a blocked thinking or a eureka moment. Moreover, as Theodore Brown points out, "metaphors based solely on embodied physical experiences no longer suffice […] and the appropriate mappings increasingly derive from social constructs, with their attendant greater complexities."[49] The *mapping* we do, whether in science or in psychology, can derive from virtual constructs such as those of mythology, literary inventions, cinematic monsters… anything that the imagination can invent. Cupid's arrows is such an example of a good metaphor: Cupid is a mythological character who sends metaphorical arrows; yet a heartbreak is often felt like a piercing of the heart. Another example is Pegasus: the winged horse never existed, yet, a horse's natural instinct is not to fight, but rather to flee, to run, to jump *as if* it had wings. In that sense, imagining a winged horse communicates something true about the nature of the horse. The horse may be like a bull in size and strength, yet, it reacts like a bird when frightened; hence a horse with wings is something that has an emotional resonance. A metaphor, like the definition Jung gave of a symbol, is false on the outside (horses don't have wings) and true in the inside (but they have flight reactions). Whenever our feelings erupt with the kind of intensity that characterizes a heartbreak, it is very healing to find the right metaphor for our particular situation, and to upgrade our imagery as the feelings change.

We easily understand why a scientist must not be too attached to a particular metaphor because when research reveals something new, the metaphor may have to change as well. I agree with Colin Turbayne when he points out that although scientific concepts are inevitably metaphoric, "there is a difference between using a metaphor and being used by it; between using a model and mistaking the model for the thing modeled. The one is to make believe that something is the case, the other is to believe it"[50]. Agreed! The same is true in formulating one's emotions in metaphors. For some individuals a heartbreak is a tsunami, and for others it is quicksand; for many it is an arrow piercing the heart, but it may also be a crucifixion, a shunning, a drowning, a choking, a killing, an hemorrhage, an amputation, a paralysis... Finding which is the right metaphor for your heartbreak is as crucial for you as for the scientist asking if proteins fold, or roll, or recoil. What is the right metaphor for your heartbreak?

In my study of heartbreak, looking at both the language of neuroscience and that of depth psychology, I found that one of the most helpful hint from Jung is this: attention to the *emerging symbols* can help the transcendent function move up, towards and into consciousness. The resolution of a heartbreak is not the re-establishment of a limbic sense of secure attachment; it is rather what Jung called the process of individuation. The pain of heartbreak can bring about a new conscious standpoint that transcends the previous opposition between love and hate, security and freedom. This new consciousness is at a higher level for a while, until the process repeats itself again, through the withdrawal of more projections, and the recognition of more contradictory impulses within oneself, leading to ever-increasing levels of consciousness.

Orient yourself: the pin on the map

The experience of bereavement has been described in countless ways which typically include a sense of radical *disorientation.* You feel lost in an unfamiliar, desolate, hostile world. You alternate between a restlessness similar to the searching behavior of the lost pup looking for its mother: "where are you, stop hiding, come back from the dead, don't disappear on me." Every white SUV car seems similar to your partner's car; he/she seems to appear at the supermarket, at the pharmacy, at the bank. I remember how, the month following the death of my father, although my rational mind knew perfectly well that he was dead and buried, each time I saw the slim silhouette of a man wearing a black Ascot cap– the kind of felt hat dad used to wear–my heart jumped *as if* he had just reappeared from the dead. This is a instinctual impulse: to search for what was lost and it creates a radical disorientation because the territory where the loss happened is nowhere and everywhere. You feel lost, disoriented, homeless, exiled, orphaned, a tourist in a hostile country with no credit card, no passport, no GPS.

The concept of *map* is one of the most often used metaphors to convey the sense that we humans, when lost in unknown territory, need the experience of others, in the form of maps, to find our way back toward the fertile land of human exchanges. Jung conceived of his psychology as a map of the psyche[51], one that millions of readers have appreciated. Philosophers, psychologists, literary geniuses, or maybe the wise old woman next door who endured a few heartbreaks, all have maps that deliver a consistent message: "you were not necessarily wrong when you were attracted to the partner, but now you are lost in a territory that you may think is love; you are mistaken, you are in the territory of compulsion. Here is a way out." There are as many maps of human relationships as there are disciplinary fields: science is mapping the neurological circuitry of love, loss, and the chemistry of depression; psychology is mapping the psychological intricacies of attachment and love addiction; songs, novels, TV series, daily gossips and anecdotal news... all show a different aspect of the vast continent of love and heartbreak.

A map is useful only if a) you are able to locate your position, and b) if you have a sense of your destination. Otherwise, if you don't know where you are, nor where you want to go, a map is useless. The problem is that a heartbreak is one of the most *disorienting* human experiences; you lost the one person who was your North star and you lost your sense of *destination*. No location and no destination! The partner was your home base, the place of the heart and of the hearth, your location in the universe, and your daily destination. *Home* is now an emotional Atlantis; and there is no other place you really want to be. In order to use a map the logical first step is to *situate* yourself, leaving for later the concern with *destination*. A psychic GPS will work only if you are fist able to inform the satellite of your situation. Orienting himself is what William did when he found the symbol of the turtle: "this is my psychic location: a dying turtle, hidden and encapsulated in myself." You need to do

[handwritten annotation: → Personify]

the same: formulate your emotions is a way that describes the psychic place you are inhabiting. It is an excellent tactic to move away from the limbic wordless moaning of the initial limbic shock; it engages your brain in neurogenesis because symbolic formulation requires the use of the most sophisticated tool that only humans have access to: language[52]. If you prefer another medium of expression (drawing, painting, playing music, dancing…), like Jung did when he did his Red Book, it works as well, as long as your formulation engages the right hemisphere of your brain (creativity and artistic expression).

Although the trauma of heartbreak is archetypal, universal, a common drama, the symbolic form it takes is unique for each person. William's symbol of the dying turtle belongs to him alone; I don't know anyone who has that exact same image. For William, finding this image was like the pin on the map that says: "you are here, this is your metaphor, you are here on the map of heartbreak: dying alone in your carapace." Somebody else may express feeling *like* an orphan, another feels *like* a fool, or *like* a beggar, or *like* a dismissed servant, or *like* a defeated general. I have interviewed individuals who felt their heartbreak was an experience that felt *like* an ambush, a test of strength, a parting of the sea, a season in hell, a glaciation, a forest fire, a tsunami, a drowning, a choking, a bankruptcy…and of course many carry the image of an arrow piercing the heart, or a knife, a bullet, a ferocious animal tearing the heart from the living body. What exactly does it feel *like* for you? Formulate it! Write it down, tell it to someone, meditate on the image, feel it in your body. A woman friend wrote that after her divorce she felt *"like a rubber band that has been stretched too often, there is no more snap in me."* A man felt *like* a retired janitor with no apartment to live in and care for; another felt *like* his psyche was hemorrhaging; a young woman wrote: "my husband was the aristocrat, and I, the hired help. I was given the pink slip, I was easily replaceable."

The next vignette is about Rita, to show how the process of formulating one's story is felt somatically; a good metaphor is an embodied image.[53] I had known Rita for four years, as a student of psychology, when I witnessed her sudden collapse. Her heartbreak was so acute that the skin on her whole body burst into a purulent eczema. She began using a technique that the Jungians call *active imagination,* which is a form of dialogue with the invisible guests living in our psyches. She did that for a month, and the more she opened her imagination, the more her skin cleared up. The following vignette summarizes the fictive conversation with her dead female ancestors, in the best tradition of active imaginaton.

RITA: A CONVERSATION WITH MY ANCESTORS

Last month, I discovered a love letter my husband wrote to another woman, confirming my suspicion. That day, I roamed the house, circling through the rooms as if to prevent death from entering the house, but death was already in the house, in my heart, in my soul, in my skin, in the form of a sudden rash. I was in a panic. I began polishing the silver, as if this would calm me. Polishing the silver turned out to be my way of calling my female ancestors: mother, grandmother, great-grandmother, and finally, my great-great grandmother Elvira, who was a wealthy hotel owner. When Elvira sold her hotel she kept the collection of silverware that was used in the hotel's dining room. I inherited it, after a long line of women, and it now fills the six glass cabinets that line the walls of my dining room. It is my collection of antiques, my only inheritance, my only luxury. As my hands were polishing those silver masterpieces, I was having a conversation with the women whose hands so often polished the same pieces.

—Have I lost him?

— Maybe he is gone forever, answered the choir of female ancestors, or maybe the affair with the other woman is just a retaliation against your busyness.

—What do you mean, busyness? He works hard, too, all day...

—Polishing the silver, hey! Always the good housekeeper. What about sexual passion? We, your female ancestors know all about your kind of busyness... we too were polishing the silver and cleaning the house and weeding the garden and always being busy while our husbands cavorted with less busy women.

— Ok, I get the message, watch me... I am going to re-seduce my husband, I'll be a geisha for a while, instead of housekeeper.

That evening, I washed the sheets on our bed, I took a long relaxing bath, I dyed and curled my hair (he likes curly blond hair), sprayed my best perfume, put a sexy nightgown on, and lighted scented candles all over the bedroom. We got in bed early and I got in beside him, naked. He remained indifferent to my nudity, indifferent to my caresses, distracted, silent. He quickly fell asleep. The next day my female ancestors were saying:

—Rita, we think your marriage is over! You created famine by giving him too little sex. We think that your husband found another fountain of joy; why would he come back to you?

—I see my mistake. I am the loveless, impeccable

housekeeper, married to the house, not the man. I don't really know how to be a lover; lovemaking is something that makes me itch! Somehow, sex annoys me, it interferes with the other things I need to do. I think I don't even know what it means to be a sexual being.

—Right. Now you know where you stand: you are somebody who does not know how to be sexual. Sex irritates you; that is why your skin is itchy!

The formulation of her story, writing this fictive dialogue as if it was her art project for the week, reading it to me and to her friends, gave her something of great value: *words to dress the wound.* Just like an artist is satisfied only when the piece of art communicates the vision, she edited that dialogue almost everyday for a week, until she felt the conversation with the ancestors had a *revelatory* quality for her. This is the true meaning of an overused, undefined and impossibly vague word: *creativity.* What does it mean, really, to be "creative" if not to *re-create* our inner reality with the best of our artistry? What is the use of creativity if not to elevate our limbic meowing, growling and howling to the level of an eternal human drama? To *esthetize* the pain, in the form of a metaphor or narrative, produces an interesting neurological impact: it intensifies the activity in the neo-cortex, a much needed distraction from the crying and obsessing. Crosswords, sudoku and mathematical puzzles also engage the neocortex, which is why they can be relaxing; but adding an artistic creation does more because it engages not only the intellect but the emotions as well. Rita's imaginary conversation with her dead ancestors had an emotional impact which doing a sudoku would not have had; it was like the pin on the map that says: you are here; discovering that sex is an irritation to you. A creative effort is needed to find the narrative that expresses your emotions with nuance and exactitude. Sometimes, reading a text written by another person gives you the metaphor you are looking for. This is one of the gift of literature: to help formulate our own inner reality. Through art and literature, we participate in the dreams of others, we feel their emotions, we visit the psychic places they visited and it helps us situate ourselves.[54] Once you have the location, you can start thinking of a destination.

CHAPTER 4

DESTINY AND DESTINATION

Others carry our souls and become our soul figures, to the final consequence that without these idols we fall into the despair of loneliness and turn to suicide. By our use of them to keep ourselves alive, other persons begin to assume the place of fetishes and totems, becoming keepers of our lives.

James Hillman[55]

One likes to believe that we can change things around us, because we cannot imagine a solution that is not the one we desire. We forget a possible favorable outcome: things don't change, but slowly, it is our desire that changes. The situation that felt unbearable becomes a matter of indifference. We could not surmount the obstacle, as we so wanted, but life forced us to take a detour; looking backward, we can barely perceive what was then felt like an obstacle.

Marcel Proust[56]

If one compares the story of a heartbreak with the history of human culture, one discovers that there seems to be only two peak experiences for which humans have been willing to die: love and freedom. A heartbreak initially deprives you of both love and a sense of freedom. Falling from the high summit of love, the most common mistake is to want to climb again to visit the peak called Love. Mistake! First, you have climb the other mountain, and explore the other peak called Freedom. But, you may ask, freedom from what? And the answer is right there in our history: freedom from the obsessive, passionate, symbiotic, neurotic elements that keep you in bondage. Human love can never be completely cleared of all its neurotic elements; such a goal is unrealistic, like wanting to find God by climbing the highest mountain; yet it is a goal we must pursue, especially when the heart is broken. When there are too many barnacles under your boat you need to scrape, clean, cut, and tidy up. Same with your heart: when there is too much obsession in the passion, the remedy is to up the level of freedom.

Break the symbiosis

We are easily seduced by the idea of a love that would encompass us totally; its pleases the frightened little mammal who whispers "keep me under your wing, in the cocoon." "Absolutely not! answers the growing human with the evolving cortex, I want to take risks, experiment, evolve...." The experience of love gives us both a safe nest to grow up or lick our wounds, and it also give us a pair of wings to leave the nest, and find identity. This fundamental contradiction, at times, feels insufferable; yet it is our most powerful agent of evolution. It is the task of a lifetime to transcend this opposition between the need for security and the need for freedom. This constant bouncing on and off our fears qualifies us as the species most capable of evolutionary leaps. "Can I do this?" Yes, let's try!" It also qualifies us as spiritual beings, because love and freedom both are victories over fear. A heartbreak starts as an experience where fear is intense while courage is in short supply. The partner is my tormentor and I want to break free, but the partner is my security and I want to get close again. It creates an exhausting push/pull: "I love you/I hate you; I need you/go away; I'll never forget you / I'll never forgive you; you hurt me/don't leave me." This tension won't go away because it is part of our neurological makeup; yet it becomes a factor of evolution (or call it: *individuation*) because it forces us, again and again, to go beyond our infantile and neurotic expectations about love.

At the beginning of a fall from Love, the wounding feels inflicted from *outside*, caused by the partner's rejection, which forces one in the passive posture of the sufferer. Passivity, so typical of the first traumatic phase of a heartbreak, is at the core of the victim archetype. It is that passivity, that *waiting for rescue* by the partner that comes to an end as you start climbing towards freedom and developing of a new network of synaptic connections. Engaging the brain with new problems, new situations, new relationships, gradually erases the addiction to the departed partner. Even in cases where the couple gets back together after a separation, the old neurotic pattern must first fade off and be replaced by a new pattern of relating. The persons in the relationship may remain the same, but their brains have to learn a new dance before reunion is possible. The formation of new synaptic connections brings a different relation to the past, the present, the future.

Although neuroscience can *explain* the process by which this kind of neuronal rejuvenation is possible, no scientist in the world can prescribe the thoughts, symbols, activities, friendships, books, movies, that will help you perform that rejuvenation. Neuroscience confirms that the synapses will get going with an opening of your imagination, with curiosity about your emotions and that of others, with a fascination for deep questions and inner adventure. A passive victim is one who is stuck in the same futile and fruitless *causal* questioning: "*why* did he/she leave me? *Why* are we always fighting about the same things? *Why* are you doing this to me?" The "why" question is a good stimulus for a scientist, who is looking for causes, but not so good for psychological rejuvenation. For one, there are an infinite number of causes which frustrate our need for one definitive answer, and, second, any reliable answer to the 'why' question would have to involve the person who broke the relationship. Your brain won't engage with such a losing strategy, but it will if, instead of *why,* you ask *who, what, how, with whom, where*. Ask yourself open ended questions:

"*who* was I becoming with my partner? (A bitch? A baby? A cash cow? A janitor? A whiny victim?). *What* can I do with my money, talent, time, that does not relate to the abandoner? *How* could I change the way I dress, work, answer the phone, talk with my friends in a way that feels fertile, fresh, fun? *What might be* the meaning of this heartbreak in the longer perspective of my life's trajectory? *With whom* could I learn to swim, sign, dance, plant a garden, do carpentry and write my memoir? *Where* can I find the best quality of silence? *Where* in my body do I feel the emotion of rage, despair, fear? Any question that can tickle your neurons into action is a good question. You can formulate the answers in writing, or explore them verbally with a friend, or with a therapist or with an imaginary companion, as in active imagination. You can express the answers in the form of a song, a poem, a novella, a renovation project, a new wardrobe, a change of professional orientation, a training, a therapy, a friendship with an unlikely type… anything as long as the answers feel *just right*, expressing a form of psychological and artistic truth. If you answer those question right, your answers should feel somehow *surprising*, which is a sign that it is an authentic response from the unconscious, as opposed to a flat egoïc invention.

Neuroscience demonstrates how the fantastic plasticity of the human neocortex is responsible for humanity's resilience. The threats from the environment are constant and ever changing and without the capacity to learn new ways our species would have disappeared. Neuroscientists all agree that ours is a learn-or-perish story. A recovery from heartbreak follows the same principle: either you transform your ways of relating to others, to yourselves and to the world, or you risk psychic stagnation, with its medical consequences. Maybe neuroscience's most important discovery, or at least the one that gives depth psychology a new relevance, is the demonstration of how, as you change your thinking, it changes your feeling. Reciprocally, if you change your feeling (through new experiences) it changes your thinking. Pathological mourning and love addiction is a *stuckness* in old feelings, old thinking, it is an engagement with ghosts, an old story going nowhere, leaving you, the protagonist, stuck in scene one, act. To turn the page and start a new chapter you must add a sense of adventure to your life, take risks, show will, and become active in your destiny.

Neuronal rejuvenation is a task that involves all three levels of the brain, each level with its set of unconscious routines –one could say, its own psychology– each with it unique organization of neurons. Let's go back to the three characters in the drama of heartbreak– the crocodile, the pup, and the wise human– and see how the neuronal re-programming of each of these character looks like in detail.

Forever keep an eye on the crocodile

> *One of the strongest lessons I learned was how to feel the physical component of an emotion. Joy was a feeling in my body. Peace was a feeling in my body. [...] I learned that I had the*

> *power to choose whether to hook into a feeling*
> *and prolong its presence in my body, or just let*
> *it quickly flow right out of me. [...] I may not*
> *be in total control of what happens to my life,*
> *but I certainly am in charge of how I choose to*
> *perceive my experience.*
>
> Jill Bolte Taylor [57].

He/she won't return your calls, won't show up, is betraying you, using you, humiliating you, making you jealous, envious, deprived, sick, lonely, angry. Or: he/she is dead, gone for all eternity, and nobody will ever replace that person, which you have turned into a god/goddess like figure. Physiologically, chemically, psychically, you *are* under attack. The reptilian brain's natural urge is either to *flee*, –for example, one can flee in an idealizing fantasy about the perfection of the departed spouse–, or to *fight* – for example, in acting out your vengeful feelings : "you jerk/bitch, you'll pay for this!" Court records are filled with stories of unrequited love that lead to revenge and murder. Statistics about domestic crime demonstrate the frequency with which rejected partners become abusive, men trying to justify their aggression with "you-made-me-hit-you" and women hiring the meanest lawyer in town: "go for the jugular, I want him utterly broke even if legal fees costs me more than the divorce settlement." Aiming for the jugular is how the reptilian brain processes the assault of rejection. Biochemically, heartbreak is an assault. If your partner died, it was evidently not a personal affront to you, yet, you are not spared the reactivity of the crocodile, even if it has no object and may be accompanied by guilt. "I need you so much; how dare you die on me!"

Just like the crocodile bites and tighten its jaws on the prey, there is a natural urge to tighten our grip on the object of our love: "you are mine, I won't let you escape." That instinctual reflex is *not* something that you can undo, precisely because it is a reflex, a default setting in the brain, part of our instinctual makeup. Nevertheless, there is a way *around* it.

First, the primitive urge must be acknowledged–"I am so angry I could kill"–. Feel the crocodile's surge of adrenaline and let it be. The Buddhists call that acknowledgement the *witness* attitude, a way of looking at your emotion as you would look at the weather. Part of witnessing is *naming* it– "here comes the croc!" This kind of discipline can limit the crocodile's reflex to the briefness that characterizes all reflexes. The best occasion to practice this discipline is with jealousy, which inevitably provokes the crocodile's reactivity. When jealousy fills your heart, feel the crocodile arising in you, don't judge its viciousness, just breathe deeply and let it be– "Whow! I am so jealous I can barely breathe!" Breathe nonetheless, deeply and slowly, because with every breath the chemical reaction lessens and soon you are past the point of automatic reactivity. Taking revenge, insulting, hitting, shouting at the partner who does not return love, all those behaviors belongs to your crocodile psychology, the kind of reaction that not only can send you to prison, but also profoundly offends the human heart! To have the *urge* to take revenge is human, but to *act* on it is too much of a concession to our reptilian brain. Revenge is not only morally offensive to our human values, it is also psychologically disastrous because it leaves us with a scarred and regressed psyche.

I am not suggesting that we should not defend our legitimate interest in a divorce settlement, but fairness is very different from vengefulness, and it implies a calm mind. Captain Ahab's obsession to take his revenge on the big white whale is one of the most powerful stories of a person indulging in a crocodile's psychology. Melville's description is beautifully precise: *"Ah, God! what trances of torments does that man endure who is consumed with one unachieved revengeful desire. He sleeps with clenched hands; and wakes with his own bloody nails in his palms*[58].

Adopt that pathetic helpless pup

So, let's assume that you have successfully learned to go beyond the crocodile urge to treat the partner as a whale of an enemy. The next task is a rewiring of the limbic connections. As opposed to reflexes, which cannot be modified, the limbic/emotional part of our brain is malleable enough to respond to "training." Animal trainers use behavioral conditioning to produce a well behaved dog, a compliant horse, a competent working elephant. The emotional brain is where the phenomenon of mirror neurons has been observed. These are neurons that fire not only as we perform a certain action but also when we watch someone else perform that action: a mother sees her baby having pleasure eating ice cream and she too feels pleasure. You see somebody laughing his heart out and you begin to smile. The discovery of this mechanism is key to the study of empathy and connectedness. It suggests that we are pre-wired for understanding others, and that we share that capacity with animals. It also suggests that the lack of this capacity may be caused by a neurological problem, as in autism, which is characterized by an incapacity to feel empathy.

The mammal-in-us does not evolve but it can be trained, and should be treated in a way that it will feel secure. As we saw earlier, the default response of our limbic brain is to fear abandonment, because an abandoned newborn mammal inevitably dies. Even if your adult self knows you are perfectly equipped to take care of your basic needs, there is still, in the folds of your brain, the memory of the earlier vulnerability. Anyone who has ever observed a lost puppy, kitten, colt, calf, has seen the best example of what psychologists call a neurotic co-dependent: whimpering, whining, helpless, a beggar for love. Our mammalian self is filled with puppy dreams of finding joy, safety, support, fun and play in a land of milk and honey, chocolate and champagne, caresses between silk sheets –all these goodies compliments of the loving partner, all free of charge. As one of my friends said: "I would love to be my dog, to have someone like me to take care of all my needs." The honeymoon usually satisfies this infantile part in us, and we enjoy, for a time, the illusion that pleasure and security are here to stay. When suddenly the milk curdles and the honey hardens because the partner betrays, dies, goes broke, works too much, lose interest, or abandons us, the panic is intense. The *implicit memory* of helplessness brings back the insecure pup who shows up *in every heartbroken individual, no exception*. This primitive self puts on an incredible show of neurotic co-dependency.

Examine your co-dependent traits

The psychiatric definition of Dependent / Co-Dependent Personality Disorder is the following: "A pervasive and excessive need to be taken care of which leads to submissive and clinging behavior and fears of separation, beginning by early adulthood and present in a variety of contexts, as indicated by five (or more) of the following: 1) Has difficulty making everyday decisions without an excessive amount of advice and reassurance from others. 2) Needs others to assume responsibility for most major areas of his or her life. 3)Has difficulty expressing disagreement with others because of fear of loss of support or approval. 4) Has difficulty initiating projects or doing things on his or her own (because of a lack of self-confidence in judgment or abilities rather than a lack of motivation or energy). 5) Goes to excessive lengths to obtain nurturance and support from others, to the point of volunteering to do things that are unpleasant. 6) Feels uncomfortable or helpless when alone because of exaggerated fears of being unable to care for himself or herself. 6) Urgently seeks another relationship as a source of care and support when a close relationship ends. 7) Is unrealistically preoccupied with fears of being left to take care of himself or herself."[59]

It is a precise and useful portrait, one that fit many persons we know, including ourselves at times. Yet the fear of being a co-dependent has created another problem: the popular illusion that one can get rid of all co-dependency and seal the heart from heartbreak. Autonomy is indeed a worthy and necessary goal in order to reach adulthood, but not if it is an unconscious defense against that co-dependent pup in us. This needy limbic self is *not only* a problem, *not only* a symptom, it is also part of the capacity to *receive*, an archetypal quality at the core of all relationships. The limbic brain is where resides our fragility and neediness but also our sensuality, playfulness, inventiveness and our capacity for attachment.

Augment attachment and lessen dependency

A child can only express: "Love me! If need be, I'll betray myself to please you. I'll deny, repress and overlook abuse." Since no parent is perfect, every child will have to do some denying and repression. Psychological theories have been found guilty of expecting of human mothers to be Mother Goddesses, forgetting that mothers have their own contradictory emotions and limitations. And so do fathers. Even the most loving and dedicated parents will somehow hurt their children. My own mother was a competent and decent enough mother who never explicitly said: "You want to eat *again*, you insatiable little bugger?" Yet, with the intensity that characterizes childhood, I remember the hunger pangs between meals (and her dislike of having to cook and serve three meals a day) as if it meant imminent famine! Maybe your father never said: "You are not a satisfactory result of my efforts... could you turn into someone else?" Yet, every child will somehow feel inadequate because, being a child means you are incompetent in more ways than one. Children love the Hansel and Gretel story because of those horrible parents who lose their kids in the woods; it symbolizes every child's instinctual threat. It is soothing to hear a story where carrying bread crumbs in your pocket will bring you right back *home*, however you define *home*.

The factor that varies from one family to the other is not so much the parental expression of frustration at their children's incessant needs, but the severity of the parental acting out on that frustration. Dangerously abusive parents are immature children themselves, and cannot put any of their needs aside to care for the vulnerable child. Some kill their child *physically*, through irresponsible actions, but many more kill or harm their child *psychically*, through lack of genuine love. It is not so much the amount of impatience or annoyance that will wound the child, but the lack of daily loving gestures. They suffer, not from what is done to them, but from what was *not given*: love, joy. Parents may be impeccable in terms of physical care and still fail to *celebrate* the joy of being and playing with their child.

Most parents avoid being murderous –although not all– but their caring, at times, will inevitably lack the compassion and joy giving quality that should define parental love. This inevitable wounding is one that no child protection agency can ever monitor.

Considering that even the good-enough family cannot spare the child a measure of panicky emotions, it entails that we all have repressed unconscious fears of abandonment. Bowlby, whose landmark studies on attachment and loss still constitutes a canon, convincingly demonstrated how the limbic need for attachment is deeper than the sexual need. Volumes have been written on his systematic observations of animal behavior and the behavior of post-war children left in orphanages. His differentiation of *attachment* from *dependency* remains an important contribution in the psychological literature. *Attachment* to the caregiver corresponds to the limbic instinctual necessity to stay close to the caregiver, to be protected from predators, to be fed and instructed. The mother has the corresponding protecting and nurturing instinct, a trait that we call *the maternal instinct* and that we share with mammals. That need for *attachment* to a significant other remains all our life, because situations of vulnerability are a constant of human life[60].

Contrary to our need for *attachment*, which never goes away, our *dependency* is expected to decrease as we grow more competent in taking care of ourselves. Most evaluations of mental health, today, are based on a similar thinking: to be healthy is to be capable of intimate *attachment* without

too much *dependency* –or co-dependency as it is now called.
Bowlby's observations on human couples convinced him
that normal healthy adults partners offer each other a basis
of security that reproduces the same maternal functions as
those carried by the mother in infancy. Healthy couples
nurture each other in a "maternal" kind of way, creating a
secure attachment, yet, with less dependency. It follows that
a loss of attachment naturally brings on a state of regression
and panic similar to the panic of the abandoned child, albeit
without the lethal risk. Theoretically, the healthy adult is
capable of taking care of his/her basic needs; however, the
loss can be so traumatic that the motivation to do so may
be lacking. Bowlby's seminal study[61] of the behavioral
consequences of abandonment and loss, both in animals and
humans, in children as well as in adults, led to his theory
about the well known theory of the four phases of normal
mourning and grieving: 1) An initial *numbing* phase; 2) a
yearning phase; 3) a phase of *disorganization* and; 4) and
a final phase of *reorganization*. His method, which is that
of ethology (the study of animal behavior), is based on the
empirical observation of the behaviors of the bereaved, from
the outside, and as such did not include the study of the brain
patterns in relation to those four phases. Nevertheless, it
showed, with an extraordinary precision of details, the extent
to which we share our limbic patterns of distress with all
mammals. If whales, dolphins, horses, dogs and cats have
heartbreak depression, you can forgive yourself some of
your love madness!

As everybody experienced childhood wounding, everybody has residual dependency issues, which flood the limbic brain when an attachment is broken. Again, it is important to understand that even if your parents excelled at parenting, you still have bundles of synapses that carry the scarring of life's inevitable challenges. Even in a picture perfect family, there can be intense fraternal rivalries, periods of grinding poverty that take all the joy away, sickness or death of a parent, abuse by a teacher or a church, incompetence of a caretaker… not to mention the wounds that come from the limitations of one's cultural milieu like "girls don't need higher education and boys don't cry." *Every* childhood is more or less traumatic, none is without wounding, and the pleasure of being alive is to discover how to get over it –by first getting under it and feeling our vulnerability. Paradoxically, a childhood that would be perfectly protected would be as great a problem as an abusive one, because it would leave a doubt about the necessity to separate, to leave the cocoon. Over-protected children sometimes grow old with an unlived life. There is a kind of theorizing about co-dependency that suggests that a healthy personality is not dependent. True: the ideal is to be attached and connected, but not dependent. Yet, this approach is guilty of reductionism when it ignores the billions of neuronal connections in the limbic brain that makes us incredibly vulnerable to loss, even if we are not pathologically co-dependent. These faulty theoretical maps have led more than one patient into a freakish emotional desert devoid of *all* relationships; like death cures sickness, one can be cured of dependency by insulating oneself against love. "I don't care for anybody and nobody cares for me. Problem solved!" I find it preferable to accept that a heartbreak is the epitome of co-dependency and to develop some compassion for this shamefully and temporarily co-dependent orphan in us. Instead of buying into the disguised moralizing of pop-psychology about co-dependency, one can develop a more intense relationship with the third character in the drama, one that has more knowledge and more education than the puppy in us: the wise human.

Becoming wiser about love

The map I am drawing here does not necessarily negate or contradict all popular theories on co-dependency, some of which I find extremely valuable. My map is not necessarily a critique of theirs, but it is one drawn from the place where neuroscience intersects with depth psychology. Neuroscience confirms two realities: the first is that our vulnerability to separation cannot be avoided, and the second is that the extreme *plasticity* of the human brain offers an extraordinary capacity to move *beyond* instinctual programming, beyond puppy love and fear of abandonment. As a archetypal psychologist might say: it is not so much the co-dependent emotions that are problematic, but rather the lack of development of the *other* archetypes. It is *not* what is *there* that creates the problem, it is what is *not there*: the adult self who could take care of the inner orphan. The inevitability of wounding means that we *all* carry, in the folds of our limbic brain, the archetype of the *orphan*; that is why it is called an archetype. Feeling orphaned is a universal experience, not one limited to kids whose parents die; the bereaved is an orphan, the immigrant in an hostile city is an orphan, the prisoner is an orphan, the sick old person dying alone in the hospital is an orphan. The limbic catastrophe is the same in all those cases. Being orphaned calls for an activation of the "higher" and uniquely human functions of the brain. That wise person in us not only perfectly capable of caring for the orphan, it is also capable of philosophical development, analytical inquiries, psychological intelligence, all in the service of a recovery. Like Jean Giono's many portraits of wise old but uneducated peasants, one should not confuse the wisdom of the soul with years of schooling, but rather with a quality of the heart and mind.

The next chapter analyses some obstacles in the way of wisdom: the wrong kind of love, the wrong kind of hope, the un-wise waiting, the immature expectations, the unwise attitudes and beliefs that turn love into a painful addiction. Wisdom, like happiness, cannot be reached directly, but indirectly, by deletion of what stands in the way. The art of becoming wiser has similarity with the art of gardening: one percent planting for ninety nine percent weeding!

CHAPTER 5

WEEDING OUT THE PROJECTIONS

Real love is wild and sad; a palpitating duo in the dark.

Bachelard[62].

Neuroscientists found themselves compelled to use a concept similar to the psychoanalytic concept of *projection* to convey the sense that our adult relationships contain memories of our earlier connections to the caretakers, in the form of neuronal circuits created in the past and still active in the brain. Those bundles of synapses fire in the present, a fact that is positive when the situation calls for responses that we learned in the past and are still are adequate for the present. For example, if your grandpa was always making humiliating comments, and you learned to keep your distance from contemptuous personalities, this lesson from the past is adequate for your present. But, the automatic firing of neurons becomes a handicap if the past acquisition has no relevance to the present. If somebody tells you that you have a piece of lettuce stuck in your mustache and you feel a terrible sense of humiliation, you are not reacting to the present but to Grandpa. It signals that *a new layer of connections* has to be added to your repertoire. When William realized he was reacting to Laura with the fear and helplessness of his childhood, it was a most precious information; it was saying: "Hey William, you need to update your wiring. You don't *need* Laura the same way you needed your Mom."

The neuroscientific perspective is consistent with the work of depth psychotherapy, inasmuch as it examines how unconscious projections are blurring our response to the present. Projections are inevitably part of the experience of falling in love, because, after all, we first learn love in the family, yet those same projections are also causing tension because the partner is *not* mom nor dad and should not carry a parental responsibility. In order to have a real connection to the partner, the mature adult has to sort out what feelings belongs to the family of origin and what belongs to the new situation. It is part of the experience of therapy to help a man discover just how much his daily projections on his wife (Madonna, whore, sister, nurse, princess, witch, lover, executioner...) come from his experience of his mother. And when a woman wonders: how is it that I turn all my lovers into my babies, the blunt answer is: projections! In neurological parlance, projections are those bundles of synapses that were established in the past and that fire up automatically in the present. Those persistent neurological networks cannot be de-activated without first resurfacing. It is the only way to become conscious of how outdated these connections are, and start updating the wiring.

It would be practical if our infantile projections emerged with one of those tags attached to electric devices: *"Warning: do not plug any new relationship in the old socket of your past wounding."* To complicate matters, the more traumatic the initial wounding, the more chances that it remains unconscious, preventing any kind of updating. A neurotic personality is one who keeps plugging actual connectors in a power outlet that delivers the energy of the infantile defenses. It produces shorts and shocks of variable intensity, which, sadly enough, feel better than no current at all. A neurotic defense often feels more comfortable than the risk of spreading our wings for the first time. Yet, in the long run, it destroys vitality.[63]

William was stunned and humiliated to discover that his fear of losing Laura had an unconscious psychic charge that came from a resurgence of his infantile panicky self. "Me? A scared, dependent, vulnerable, pre-verbal, helpless, clingy, needy, unconscious person? Impossible!" The discrepancy between his adult competent self– not to mention his recent Ph.D. in psychology– and the regressed needy child was a crucial insight. He intellectually understood, and more importantly, he *felt, experienced* and *re-lived,* in full cinematographic precision, how his panic at losing Laura was the same he experienced, repeatedly, when his socially busy mother would look at him as if he were a mild nuisance. He physically *felt* how terrified he had been of her cold, almost indifferent rejecting attitude. His defense, first as a child, then as an adult, had always been to leave any relationship first. Defense mechanisms are as varied as the forms a heartbreak takes; this individual will become a pleaser while another will react by becoming aloof, or dominating, or co-dependent. The idiosyncratic *style* in which you defend yourself is not as important as the fact that a defense mechanism quickly becomes a waste of psychic energy. Think of your preferred defense mechanism as a familiar pair of deforming glasses, so familiar, you forget you have them on. A defense mechanism starts as a good enough management of psychological resources, a coping strategy, which is why it is called a *defense* mechanism– it protects the vulnerable psyche against dangerous emotional overload. As children, we survive our vulnerability by *not* becoming aware of any fact that would be unbearable.

A very common example of the necessity of defense mechanism is a child's behavior at a mother's or a father's funeral: young children do not – and *should not–* experience the full impact of such a loss. I remember a five year old boy, whose father had suddenly died; he behaved as if not concerned with all the fuss and the tears around him, staying prudently away from his distressed mother, running around the buffet served after the funeral, tasting everything as if it was his birthday party; he was disconnected, aloof and emotionally unreachable. It would be overwhelming for the psyche of a young child to realize the amplitude of such a loss; hence the brain offers the option to deny, disconnect, repress, ignore. Like a power bar with a surge protector, the psyche of a child automatically disconnects if the charge is dangerously high. Adults do it too, although they can handle higher charges.

A defense mechanism becomes troublesome when the child's worldview blurs the vision of the adult. For example, the child might have tought: "I was a really bad boy yesterday, and mommy died that day" . This kind of faulty association might literally remain inscribed in the folds of the child's brain, and later manifest in the form of neurotic guilt. The grown-up man who discovers that he has always equated being a bad boy with killing his mother, might finally understand how, each time he hears the slightest criticism from his wife, he overreacts. "My wife asks me, with some measure of reproach, why I keep forgetting to take out the garbage and I hear: you are bad and it is killing me." This kind of reaction is the essence of a neurotic projection, based on an outdated bundles of synaptic connection, firing as in the past. Becoming conscious of his projections from the past had great value for this man; he saw how his adult relationship with his wife *contained* not only the past guilt, but the potential for updating. As a mature man, he could finally understand what the child could not: "mom didn't die because I was a bad boy, but because she had cancer." What a relief! When that insight occurs, the adult is ready to drop the neurotic defense, and respond with a more adapted behavior. "Oh, yes, the garbage, thanks for the reminder, I keep forgetting!" The trigger that brought out the outdated synaptic connection has been deactivated.

Such unconscious responses, which provided the bread and butter for psychoanalysts and therapists for the past century, are now described by neuroscience as a bunch of *pre-wired synaptic connections ready to fire*. This kind of unexamined responses, coming from a lesson we learned in the past, can be life-saving, when they are adapted to the situation.

Many of our daily routines are accomplished without conscious control. They stem from what neuroscientists call the non-conscious, implicit domain which is also called procedural memory. For example, driving home in your car does not demand that you be conscious of every gesture you make to navigate your way home. The notion of a defense mechanism is different; it is grounded in the dynamic unconscious of psychoanalysis. Yet, when the threat takes a different form but our response does not, it becomes what psychologists call a neurotic pattern.

Keep your heart open

Love provokes an inner expansion that, in turn, augments the capacity to feel the beauty of the outer world; lovers have memories of admiring a starry sky, as if looking up at the sky for the first time; or of tasting food as if the number of taste buds had suddenly multiplied; of making love as if for the first time. In love the capacity to feel is amplified. The manner in which the perception of the outer world and the experience of the inner world are neurologically connected explains how, as love expands the inner realm, it also provokes a multiplication of the neurons that allow us to perceive the outer world. In the euphoric period of falling in love, this expansion is easy and pleasurable; like a child learning language, lovers quickly learn many new behaviors that solidify their bond. The loss of the beloved is the reverse experience: your heart is still wide open, and your neurons are firing, but that openness of the heart is now felt as torture, because the connection to the Beloved is broken. Your vulnerable heart won't stop feeling, won't close, it remains painfully open because the neurons that connected you to your partner are still active in your brain. You can't help wanting the partner to come back, and literally reconnect you to the world.

At the time when love was plentiful, even mundane tasks had an amplified meaning –cooking, fixing things in the house, choosing the new color to repaint the walls, mixing cement to built a little fountain in the garden, teaching the child to use the digital camera to send grandpa an email ... it all made sense because it expressed the loving connection. Love reveals what a philosopher might call the *transcendent quality* of human life. It brings an accentuation of your being, like a number squared; it is the revelation of something beyond the evidence of the senses. Love grounds you in the concreteness of daily life, while at the same time reflecting the infinity of the cosmos in the inner sanctum of the heart. When the purveyor of love abandoned you, all the bundles of synapses that connected you to that person remained active, but with no response, creating a situation of emotional inertia. The lack of echo is experienced as the inner abyss in which you fall. The bitterness of mourning has *the same amplifying power* as had the sweetness of love, but in reverse. The daily routine that felt so meaningful now feels meaningless, because it reveals the loss.

We all readily admit that both the bitter and the sweet are part of the love potion, but until we are forced to drink the potion to the dregs, we rarely take the time to analyze what causes that bitter aftertaste.

Taste the bitter

Staying with the darkness allows something to happen that escapes us if we are hasty. If we resist our natural tendency to take flight before painful experiences, we can descend into the dark aspects of the unconscious, which is necessary if we are to make contact with what Goethe calls "infinite nature." Turning toward such darkness requires a willingness to stay with suffering and to make a descent into the unconscious.

Stanton Marlan[64]

No one should deny the danger of the descent, but it can be risked. No one need risk it, but it is certain that some will. And let those who go down the sunset way do so with open eyes, for it is a sacrifice which daunts even the gods. Yet every descent is followed by an ascent; the vanishing shapes are shaped anew, and the truth is valid in the end only if it suffers change and bears new witness in new images, in new tongues, like a wine that is put into new bottles.

Carl Jung[65]

If your parents were competent enough, you hold the cellular memory of having been a little person whose needs for comfort and security were more or less met; your limbic brain developed normally, and you grew into a relatively secure child. Yet, with adolescence, a terrible contradiction developed between the limbic part of your brain, which still depended on your family for love and support, and your specifically human cortex, whose function, among others, is to help you become independent of your caregivers. Without that urge to become independent, you would never have been able to separate, to take leave. The development of human culture is based upon that exclusively human capacity to cut ourselves from the security of the pack, in order to innovate, take risk, try new ways. This impulse to explore and experiment explains why adolescence is such a difficult time. Without this human capacity to leave the security of family, tribe, church or country, there would be mostly repetition of the same, from one generation of humans to another– no art, no science, no evolution in our code of law, no quest for a personal identity. The fact that we can risk leaving behind the identity given by the family, has allowed our species to develop our unique cognitive abilities, to acquire control over our conditions of living and to survive our ever changing ecosystem. The way we eat, work, relate, administer justice, educate our youths, develop new technologies, do commerce… all depend on our capacity to *invent, control, adapt, evolve.* A house heated by a central furnace and a thermostat in every room in a beautiful example of our capacity to *control* an environment that is too harsh for our vulnerable human bodies. Art and science, technology and commerce, medicine and language... all depend on this capacity to separate from the pack.

A situation of bereavement recapitulates the basic challenges faced by all humans, at all times; your emotional niche has been destroyed and it is a threat that signals to your brain that it is time to *invent, control, adapt, evolve* in order to survive. If we could look back at our biography with an extra lucid mind, we could retrace all the threats we faced in our lifetime by the lessons we learned, or failed to learn. Unfortunately, we are not necessarily aware of those lessons; they are all there, in the folds of the brain in the form of a bunch of synaptic connections that are expressed in the forms of preferences, habits and fears. The difficulty is that those connections are, to use the big U word, *unconscious.*

Uncover pre-verbal memories

I have a friend, a weather journalist, who likes to tell his story using the words of neuroscience because he does not know any of the vocabulary of depth psychology. His formulation is the best example I could find of how neuroscience redefines the psychoanalytic concept of the unconscious and permeates the cultural discoure.

MY LIFE IN A COPTER

I come from a family of mountain dwellers in the Alps. The older members of my family are all familiar with the sound *of a coming avalanche, a sound that provokes in them an instinctual (reptilian) state of alarm. In fact, anybody in the village who ever experienced the death threat of such a situation reacts to that sound by an alarm of the whole involuntary neurovegetative system. It is what behaviorists call a conditioned reflex and what neuroscience calls a trigger of the flight reaction: here is an enemy too big to fight, time to flee! And because the adults around me are humans, and not animals, they could imagine ahead, see they would be trapped in the avalanche (envisioning the future) which makes them call for help (rational judgment) on their phones (technology). When a rescue helicopter arrives, the young members of our community modeled their behavior after the educated adults (transmission of culture).*

I was one year old when that situation arrived, and had not yet been conditioned to feel instinctual alarm at the sound of an avalanche. Soon after this experience, my parents divorced and I left the Alps with my mother, to live in Canada.

The sound of an avalanche, to the baby I was when I heard it for the first time, would have been equal to any other non-threatening sound, like that of the washing machine or that of the snow blower. Just a sound. But I heard it in my mother's arms, who was in a state of panic like everybody around her, waiting for rescue from an helicopter, outside in the snow. Two neuronal associations were created in

*my brain: one that says here is a sound (avalanche)
and a smell (the smell of snow), that means "danger."
And another association that says: here is a sound
(the copter motor) that means safety. I was unaware
that such a bundle of synapses had remained in my
brain. I was told the story of that avalanche at fifty,
until then I never knew what motivated my choice of
becoming a weather journalist, who spends all his
working hours in a helicopter.*

My friend has a neurologically correct story: a child's
limbic capacity is developed enough to register mom and
dad's panic, but until around eighteen months, because
language is not yet developed, the child cannot interpret
the *context* (i.e. the full story going on around him). A
child is a limbic genius when it comes to *feeling* either
the panic signals or the soothing signals coming from the
adults. When the rescue helicopter came in, although its
motor made a much louder noise than the avalanche, my
friend's infantile brain taught him: trust mom, who trusts
the rescuers, who trust the copter, but don't ever trusts the
sound of an avalanche, or the smell of snow. Any incident
that happens before the hippocampus (part of the limbic
brain) is fully developed, makes the stocking of *explicit
memory*[66] impossible and is responsible for *infantile
amnesia*. As language develops, the child starts being able

to remember the event, the context and the time sequence and now has *words* to tell the story. The retrieval of such memory is sometimes called *episodic memory*, or *autonoetic memory* (i.e. knowing that I know). Some authors also refer to episodic memory as *narrative memory* to point at the fact that it is a form of memory which includes a time sequence. For example, if you tell the factual details of a car accident, you will remember that it took place last week, mid-morning, there was a sedan car on the left... a red truck coming from the right, rain and fog...a frontal impact... . you organize the events in a time sequence in a *story* of the accident. I find it interesting that the act of recollecting and reflecting upon one's past is neurologically similar to the act of *anticipating* one's future. We don't use the word memory when imagining our future, but rather words like imagination, day dreaming, planning, fantasizing, yet, it is neurologically similar operation to reminiscing.[67] By contrast to the *autonoetic* (I know that I know) memory, for which we know we are in the act of recollecting a story, a *noetic* (knowing) memory is one where we don't need to recall the past to remember something that has become a semi-conscious routine, like reaching for your car keys in your purse or driving your car from work to home.

The capacity for narrative autonoetic memory develops along with the ability to use language; before we have words, the trauma, and the positive or negative lesson we learned from it, is inscribed in the brain but you cannot verbalize it. My friend was not told the story of the avalanche until he was fifty years old. The fact that the smell of snow triggered an automatic reaction of unease had remained an unexplained mystery. He never could explain his nervousness whenever he visited his father's family in the Alps. He never knew why he so wanted to become a weather reporter, spending all his working hours in a helicopter; and he never knew what motivated his choice to live in California. When told of the avalanche episode, a new awareness was possible. This example does not suggest that the unconscious is an anatomical structure, but rather that what depth psychologist conceive as an unconscious reaction is *a memory without a context*. A heartbreak is an experience where the pre-verbal fear of abandonment is re-activated. Abandonment in adult life sends an alarm to the brain that is of the same nature as a threat from nature. The message is not "ALERT: Avalanche Coming" but rather: "ALERT: Loss of Love Coming." The brain remembers: loss of love, for the little mammal, means pain and a lethal risk. Although the adult rational brain knows that abandonment does not run the same risk as in the past, there is a sub routine on the hard disk of our memory that generate a sense of acute panic. To delete this fear-generating automatic alarm system –which is a standard attachment to all human psyches – you need to understand how it works.

De-activate the fear-generating software

The abandonee knows very well in whose arms he/she would want to take shelter, but that person is both the attacker and the rescuer, both the avalanche and the copter. "You are the one I need, and the one who tortures me." That is quite a puzzle for the neocortex! Hospital emergencies are filled with patients whose symptoms express a panic similar to that of the wolf separated from the pack, or that of a person shunned by the whole clan. The symptoms that brought William to the hospital emergency room are called: *stress cardiomyopathy*. Another name for it is: *apical ballooning syndrome*, which is described as a condition of the heart that happens when the brain, following an emotional trauma, releases chemicals into the bloodstream that cause rapid and severe heart muscle weakness (*cardiomyopathy*)[68]. The symptoms are very similar to patients having a heart attack. Since a heartbreak often provokes that reaction, it became known as the *broken heart syndrome*. This somatic reaction was for William the second signal from his brain, sounding the same alarm as when he came at Laura's door and she accused him of intrusion on her privacy, and showed no compassion for his distress. The second time, the alarm was sounding with more urgency: "How many times must I repeat that you have to *detach or die*?" At the hospital's emergency clinic, William was informed that he was not having a heart attack, but that he was suffering from *stress cardiomyopathy* and he received sedation which temporarily helped him. Dr. Rich, the cardiologist from the Mayo clinic who educated the public about this syndrome has this to say: "apical ballooning syndrome (ABS) is a unique reversible cardiomyopathy that is frequently precipitated by a stressful event, and has a clinical presentation that is indistinguishable from a myocardial infarction. [...] The term *Broken Heart Syndrome* may not be the best name for this syndrome, as one typically thinks of a broken heart as something that occurs after receiving a Dear John letter, rather than something that happens after seeing a loaded .44 magnum shoved in one's face. Nonetheless, this terminology has resulted in lots of publicity, and the knowledge of this new syndrome consequently has been rapidly and widely disseminated. And that widespread awareness is good. The symptoms of BHS are so severe that it is nearly inconceivable that anyone who develops it will fail to seek medical help[...]."[69]

In a severe heartbreak, the fear of abandonment is amplified to an unbearable level by the fact that there is no access to the comforting arms of the trusted caregiver, because that person is also the one responsible for the abandonment. This impossible contradiction summarizes the tragic paradox of human relations: "I need you, I resent you for it." When the partner is all, being rejected or abandoned by that most important person breaks our trust in all of humanity; we feel as if dropped by the mother, cursed by the father, snubbed by the sister, betrayed by the brother, delivered to the enemy by the friend. Our footing is no longer sure on the earth and the ego-shattering immensity of that loss sends us into a spin of denial: we refuse to take in what is happening, we cannot accept that the partner is leaving, or choosing somebody else, or gone forever with no coming back from death. The experience of heartbreak is called *archetypal* because all humans, despite their talent, beauty, fame, intelligence, experience helplessness and panic when love is denied.

I knew a woman whom everyone thought of as the ultimate image of success: bright, sexy, mature, charming, competent, a warm and decent women whom everyone admired and loved. She fell in love with a narcissistic guy, who betrayed her regularly and almost absentmindedly. Her friends, including myself, all thought: how could *she* (such a loving and wonderful person) let *him* (such an immature selfish Jerk) break her heart? How is it possible? I had a similar, but reversed surprise with a student, who, at twenty seven, was considered by the others in the class as an immature self-centered playboy, who boasted of having used every woman who ever approached him. One day he expressed his love and admiration to an older woman in the classroom, and found himself politely dismissed. After a few unsuccessful attempts to get her attention, he went home and committed suicide, leaving behind a love letter to her. We were all stunned! He had a heart after all? It was obviously a neurotic infatuation, because he barely knew this woman, but a heartbreak based on an illusion of love is not necessarily easier to get over than a heartbreak based on "true love" —— a concept to be examined in a later chapter. In both the case of the brilliant woman betrayed by an immature partner, and the egoistic student rejected by a woman he barely knew, *something* in the rejection was insufferable, unbearable.

That *something* is an unconscious reactivation of the early terror of abandonment; somehow it felt easier to commit suicide than to go through that pain a second time. Hence the necessity of undoing the early equation where abandonment equals death.

Stop trying to repair the past

Our natural egocentricity makes it difficult for us to accept our mortality; we all know death is inevitable, but when it comes to *our* death, it becomes a personal tragedy. That same natural egocentricity makes us confuse love, the impersonal infinite principle –as impersonal as life and death– with the *person* of the partner, with whom we experience our breakdown. Your beloved is mortal, finite, limited, unique and eventually replaceable, while the principle of love is eternal, infinite, essential, cosmic and irreplaceable. The differentiation between Love, –a divinity, really– and the partner –just a person–, is not easy for the psyche, but it is one of the keys to freedom.

For the ancient Greeks, falling in love turns you into a fool, but refusing love makes you an even bigger fool because it deprives you of the only way to experience the full extent of human emotions. Greek wisdom suggests that it is preferable to get drunk on the love potion rather than remain sober and half alive. Theirs was a Dionysian and Aphrodisian mentality. One of the many paradoxes of psychic life, maybe the most interesting one, is that love hurts –those damned arrows– and love teaches; love heals and love wounds, hence the necessity to befriend the tears that make us wiser.

We confuse love with the person of the partner not only because of our inevitable egocentric consciousness, but also because our brain analyzes the present with the lessons from the past, and in the past, the caregivers were our first divinities, absolutely non-replaceable. That feeling is later transferred on the person of the partner, and he/she appears with the halo of the original divinity. "Ah! It is You, Sweet Lover. I remember how it felt to have my every need met; come fill my heart, I've missed you." When the partner suddenly fails to deliver the honey, the shock is intense: "How dare you drop me so cruelly! I need you so completely." The brain not only confuses the lover with the unconscious mother complex, but often creates a split between the Good Mother and the Terrible Mother: "Your love feels safer, more generous, more joyous than what I got from Mother; you are what I craved and never got." As long as the partner gives us the honey, which is the positive side of the mother archetype, we are in the honeymooner's paradise. It feels nice for a time, yet when the part that psychoanalysts call the 'idealized transference' is shattered we find ourselves in hell.

There is a logic in every feeling, a *psycho-logic*, and there is a logic too in our expectation that love should repair past wounding; it makes sense because love *does* have that potential. Every deep loving relationship has the power to heal. "My mother thought I was ugly, but you say I am beautiful and my heart believes you. Oh Joy!" Yet, in the psycho-logic of heartbreak, there is one essential condition for love to work its healing magic: *the original wounding first has to be made conscious.* It happened for William when he *recognized* the origin of the feeling of having to beg for Laura's affections, as a feeling he first experienced with his mother. He *saw through*[70] the actual grief, as a wound from the past; it was his first step toward retracting his projections, which is at the core of the process of developing the wise adult in us.

When the need to repair becomes too much of a burden, the relationship is bound to break down. The partner cannot help feeling: "I am not the one who broke your spirit, cut your wings, said you were ugly, stupid, and a loser, why should I be the one to suffer the consequences of your brokenness? Why should I atone, expiate, compensate, repair, for damage I did not cause? You are not with me in *our* story, you are engaged with the villains of your past." Such a relationship is insulated from the reality of the present, and it becomes too rigid to survive. Any relationship, including friendship, if it is in repair mode most of the time *has* to break down. The individual too unconscious of the past wounding is basically saying: "Give me, give me more, give me always, because I did not receive enough in the past." We all have had the experience of crossing out somebody from our list of friends because there is never any possibility of reciprocity. The breakdown of those relationships is a response from nature that delivers the most crucial truth for us to evolve: the past, because it is past, can never be fixed! However, the wounding from the past *can* be transformed into something that enhances emotional intelligence, once we accept that although the past itself cannot be changed, we can.

Some heartbreaks are saying: "When will you understand that you will *never* have the loving, competent, warm-hearted nurturing mother you so needed as a child?" Others are saying: "When will you get over the fact that your daddy was, and will remain, for all eternity, a lousy alcoholic bum incapable of loving?" And all are saying: "Nobody is asking you to demean or forget your beloved, but to open up, live and learn the world anew."

Something is wrong when a woman spends a lifetime complaining of not finding the partner who would love her the way she would like to be loved; something is off when a widower raises the bar of possible partners to fit the idealized dead spouse. Again, there is a logic: no amount of loving by an actual person can ever fill the abysmal pit of cravings that belongs to the child we once were. The *unconsciousness of the lack, not the lack itself*, has created the unrealistic expectations, the repeated failures, the gloominess of permanent disappointment which invariably leads to the loveless isolation that the person is complaining about. These individuals have failed to hear their disappointments and heartbreaks as a call from nature; they have refused to evolve beyond the immature dream of being saved, healed, taken care of (financially, emotionally, socially, intellectually, physically...).

A fifteen year old girl might daydream that the perfect soul-mate is just around the corner, and that once he shows up, he will offer her identity and security, motherlove and motherland, fatherlove and fatherland, money and honey, but it is a tragedy when it defines the adult personality. In a culture where the dominant values are around money, fame, sex and power, those unconscious expectations often translate in those same terms; yet even an abundance of money, fame, sex or power will fail to deliver healing to an unconscious wounding. In every heartbreak, the potential for evolution is immense: it can shatter for good the dream of a symbiotic relationship and put an end to the idealized projections. As Jung described it, the process of individuation is as much a separation from one's cultural conditioning as it is a unification with the deeper aspects of one's psyche.[71]

CHAPTER 6

ANGER

William woke up one morning ready to use his anger as a sword, to cut himself loose and find resolution. He wrote this email to Laura:

TERMINUS

For ten months, I have been waiting for a clarification that you won't or can't give me. When you severed the sexual bond between us, you asked if we could remain friends. My answer today is this: maybe! But first I need a clean cut, to put an end to my hope, and to cool my sexual desire for you. These feelings have to die off before I can be your friend.

I have completed the cycle of analyzing and figuring "us" out. I have communicated all I needed to express and this is truly my last conversation about "us" and my last email to you. I am grateful for all the love and immense joy that I experienced with you. After a year or two of mourning you as my lover, I

> *may be able to be your friend again, I won't deny the deep affection I have for you. Life is unpredictable, and often surprising. But for now, I want a complete severance until I get myself back. Please respect my silence; don't call, don't email and don't show up. I have changed my phone number, rented my apartment and I am leaving for a year's sabbatical.*

When William wrote that final email, he had been hooked on hope for almost a year. All that time, Laura kept telling William she still loved him but also loved Jack. She was adamant that she could not be sexual with both. It is only when William's anger swell into a tsunami that he saw how Laura's confusing ambivalence was for him a repetition of his experience with his own mother, who never could come up with a clear choice, a clear emotion and a clear commitment about being a mother. William's mother was ambivalent, covert, withdrawn, aloof. Laura's natural ambivalence made William regress to being the neglected boy of that ambivalent mother. His anger was a useful, clean, legitimate reaction. The email he sent Laura was not an attack on her, it was an attack on the element, in love, that kept him in bondage. The anger broke his shackles; he took his distance, he became active instead of reactive. Taking his leave from Laura gave him the energy to open another chapter in his story.

Anger as cure for co-dependency

We have seen how heartbreak brings out traits of *co-dependency*: as long as you remain passive and re-active, you have no access to your anger. A co-dependent is the same thing as what the AA movement has defined as an "enabler"– somebody who supports the addiction of the partner by entertaining the fantasy that the partner will change. "I am sure this time he/she will keep his/her promise" is the kind of delusion one hears again and again from an enabler, in support of the status quo. Before psychologists began putting clinical labels on personality traits, "enabling" was called by many other names: weakness of character, credulity, maternal over-protection, love madness, ignorance, unreason… all of which point at an incapacity to express anger and look at things as they are– a tough task for any of us! The notion of co-dependency has expanded in popular psychology to mean almost any behavior that is purely reactive as opposed to active. A heartbreak first makes you as impotent as a declawed animal, which means that you must re-learn to access it. Anger contains energy; it leads to action, as opposed to reaction. All mammals are equipped with a capacity to express anger, as warning to the intruder.

In humans, anger is a more complex reaction, because *expressing* anger (as opposed to simply *feeling* it) can be morally wrong, which does not mean that anger per se is wrong; anger is a neurological reality that cannot be denied and it is necessary for survival. What makes us mistrust our anger is the fact that it is also the source of sociopathic behaviors. The psychologist Charles Stewart[72] did a detailed psycho-social analysis of young mass murderers and he concludes that it is never anger per se that is the trigger in such tragedies, but what he calls an *eclipse of the life instinct*. His research shows that it takes a combination of the following four conditions for anger to turn into murderous acting out: 1) *Social isolation*, which Stewart defines as a lack of "affective dialogues framed by *Interest* and *Joy.*" 2) *Dissociation of the personality*, which is the clinical phenomenon that takes everybody by surprise when the decent and apparently nice guy next door turns out to be a serial killer. 3) *Chronic unbearable affects* such as panic, terror, or a sense of falling into an abyss, happening everyday, to the point where it destroys the desire to live. 4) *Possession by affect*, such as intense jealousy, or obsessive desire for revenge with no capacity to gain any distance from one's emotions (what I call the crocodile psychology….). These four conditions for the emergence of lethal behavior have more to do with the *absence* of positive human emotions rather than the *presence* of anger. Not all individuals who experience social isolation, dissociation, unbearable affects and possession by affect will shoot in the crowd before turning the gun on themselves, but, according to Stewart, all of those who do, were experiencing all four factors. Stewart concludes they could have been helped by a proper intervention, relieving pressure at any of those points. The pathology described by Stewart should not be confused with a healthy expression of anger.

As Buddhism teaches, there is no need to *hate* the attacker to defend oneself; moral restraint does not mean one should tolerate abuse. If a thief breaks into your house in the middle of the night, anger will produce the needed adrenaline without the need to hate the thief. There is such a thing as "healthy anger" and it is part of the ecology of human relations.

Anger and leave-taking

Co-dependents have no access to the energy of anger which is why their therapy always involves an awareness of their repressed anger. When a parent, a boss, a teacher shames you unfairly, a lover betrays you, a friend talks behind your back, a business partner steals your profit, a politician distorts the truth and wastes your tax money, a delinquent scratches the paint on your car... anger is a legitimate response. *Feeling* the anger and being open to the information it contains is a healthy component of any relationship. Being informed by your anger is especially crucial in a heartbreak because it contains the energy *to take leave*, as William did when he sent Laura the final email. Your brain interprets the trauma of abandonment just like a physical attack and denying that such an attack causes anger contradicts the instincts. To avoid the gluey passivity of co-dependency, let this anger rise to your awareness; don't judge it, and use its valuable energy.

The crucial ethical point is that anger against your partner *does not legitimize retaliation in any form whatsoever.* The partner, contrary to the business partner who steals your benefits, or to any other kind of crook, does not *owe* you love, and you don't have any rights on the *person* of the partner. Love between adults, unlike other aspects of our social contract, is not a due. Even the marriage contract, which includes the promise of fidelity and devotion to the needs of the partner, cannot promise desire nor love. You can sue the crook and catch the thief but you cannot sue the partner for taking back her/his heart. Once you start shouting insults you know that your angry energy needs to be re-directed. Although there is no limit to how much anger you can *feel*, there are moral and legal limits on how much anger you can *express*, which is why the law protects its citizens with the possibility of obtaining a restraining order against an infuriated ex-partner. When the partner *takes back* his/her heart, there is no theft because the heart is free. The partner did not steal anything: your heart is still yours, if you care to pick it up from the trash bin, dust it, and teach it to use that anger in a constructive way, to grow wings instead of fangs.

We have seen how abused children learn to *dissociate* (deny, repress, forget, ignore…) from their anger because of their total dependence on the caregiver. Expressing anger creates an insufferable contradiction between "Mommy, I hate you" and "Mommy, I so need you." Whenever anger is denied because we don't have the means to be independent, it infantilizes us.

In every heartbreak, there are moments when the clash between love and anger reaches uncomfortable heights and the psyche defends itself with dissociation: "Me? angry? no way! I just want him/her back" In a pathologically co-dependent adult, this defense has shaped the personality from infancy, whereas in the heartbroken individual the resolution sounds like the title of an old movie classic: *The Return of the Repressed*. The repressed anger must be allowed to speak its truth again for the heart to heal. How could you *not* be angry at being abandoned, rejected, betrayed, shunned, snubbed, ignored? But how *could* you be angry when you were brought to your knees begging for his/ her love? Resolving this paradox is the antidote to *clinging*, a clinging that comes from a memory of having no other choice but to depend on the caregiver. No child can move out of a position of passive recipient of love because a child is not free. The corollary is this: as long as you remain on your knees, waiting for Beloved, you remain a child.

Fear of distance and fear of fusion

With the onset of adolescence, to the infantile fear of being abandoned is added the opposite fear: that of losing our newly found independence. Every adolescent is caught between the fear of *losing* ("Mom please do my laundry" or "Dad please don't cancel the credit card') and the fear of *fusing* ("Don't control me, let go of me, I need to become myself"). In adult relationships we re-visit that same conflict; at times we feel that the partner is too distant and at other moments that the partner is too close for comfort. This constant balancing between closeness and distance can be almost effortless when the relationship is functional, but in heartbreak the abandonee is stuck at the pole of wanting more closeness while the abandoner wants escape. With that kind of polarized positioning, the more you insist on closeness, the more the partner wants to escape, which is logical, because your clingy attitude does not communicate love, but panic. You re-enact not only the infantile fear of abandonment, but also the adolescent drama of "I still need you and I resent you for it." The resurgence of both the childhood dependency and the adolescent's fear of fusing explains your regressed co-dependent attitudes, which are not the most attractive aspect of your personality!

The proper use of anger: activation of your decision

There is, in all complaining, a subtle
dose of revenge.

Nietzsche[73]

Anger is the ally you need to detach, separate, take leave. To be useful, anger must first be purified of hysterical or abusive indulging. Anger cannot be in the service of envy, jealousy or revenge; it cannot serve greed, nor can it be paired with reproaches and demands. Anger is the antidote to co-dependency only if it is not confused with complaining, whining or festering resentment. To find examples of "healthy anger" I asked my graduate students to tell me their stories about positive expressions of anger. A young man came up with the story of his great-grandmother, who, fifty years ago, confided to her rabbi that she was limiting births with the calendar method. He shamed and shunned her. My student's grandmother, as a heartbroken young mother with four kids and an alcoholic husband, was so angry that she simply disobeyed. She not only continued to use contraception, she obtained a divorce and moved to a bigger city, to find work. The pain of having been shunned from her immediate community and abused by her husband, turned into a magnificent fury, an almost inexhaustible power source. From being a frustrated, exhausted, housebound wife and mother, she evolved into an indomitable women's rights activist and later, after going back to the local university, she became a beloved professor of history. In her sixties, she became the mayor of the small city she had moved to, at the time of her divorce. That woman, says her grandson, is still, at eighty, a beacon of compassion, her anger ready to surface when she sees injustice. It was anger that first gave her the boost of energy that propelled her out of a backward milieu and into a life of devotion to the values she believed in. She used that energy to *destroy* something (her submission to a an oppressive credo) and to *build* something (her self, her career and a future for her four kids). Hers was a personal revolt against the husband, the rabbi and the milieu, yet it fueled her revolt against collective values she believed were spiritually wrong. Anger gave her the courage to take her distance from her milieu, and the courage to act.

Take your distance

You think that I can't live without your love,
You'll see. You think I can't go on another day.
You think I have nothing without you by my side,
You'll see. Somehow, some way. ....
(Madonna, from the lyrics of the song: You'll See.)

The rush to move to a new relationship often covers a denial of anger, and of the emotional meaning of the loss. It isn't a real move of the psyche, it is agitation. Mourning calls for introversion, silence, solitude, in contrast with business values which demand of workers to be minimally disturbed by grief. Reclusion, so crucial to heal the heart, is counter productive from a business point of view, but necessary for rejuvenation. Gone is the time when Freud in *Mourning and Melancholy,* could insist on the need to properly mourn not only the loss of our loved ones, but as well the loss of country, loss of freedom, loss of faith, loss of an ideal. Freud's argument, that failure to mourn develops into what he called a *melancholic depression,* is not very popular nowadays, although research in psychosomatic symptoms shows plenty of evidence that Freud was right. The injunction to *move on* and *get over it*, creates a culture where people keep *moving on* so much and so fast, they end up withdrawing their interest from the world, a dizzy fixation on emptiness. Depression as we all know, is epidemic, but the connection with *un-mourned losses* is rarely explored. We also know that depression is a state where anger has been suppressed.

137

There are two avenues to a proper mourning, which may at first appear to be contradictory, but are in fact a natural pair of opposites that complement each other: solitude and reaching out. On the one hand, it is crucial to establish new connections, to find a support group, to develop new interests, to make new friends, travel or try new things, even if at first it feels like an effort. On the other hand, it is as crucial to find moments and places where one can *retreat* in silence and solitude, and mourn. Aloneness and isolation (felt as the painful unavailability of the beloved) must be replaced by an appreciation for *solitude*, which is a very different concept than isolation. Solitude offers the silence and tranquility needed to turn inward. Bossuet, the great preacher at Louis the XIV court was wrong about many things – most of all about the divine right of kings– but one can appreciate how he differentiated between different kinds of silence: 1. the silence of concentration on a task; 2. the silence that is inspired by prudence; 3. the silence of *patience* when experiencing contradictions. Adding to his list, one can imagine many more categories of silence: the silence of the media (go on TV diet); the silence of the body (as in fasting); a cat-like silence (tip-toeing away from agitation); the silence of the grass growing or the silence of snow falling (sit down and look at nature), whatever calms you. The silence of mourning does not mean no sound, it means you stop *emitting* and start *listening* to your heart with the kind of *patience* that Bossuet relates to the silence of contradictions. You stop your inner dialogue with Beloved, stop the arguing with yourself, stop broadcasting your distress – even to yourself– until there is a relaxation of the suffering ego. It hurts to be abandoned and it hurst to fail at keeping the other by our side. The ego needs calm to digest its colossal failure.

Most spiritual disciplines recognize the benefits of a silent retreat to bring peace, rest, rejuvenation. Each tradition offer techniques to quiet the mind (prayer, song, meditation) and to rest bodily functions (fasting, yoga). One doesn't need to be a religious person to benefit from those traditions. The Ancient Greeks had the concept of *incubation*, which meant a kind of introversion that was at the core of all healing processes. The patients came to the healing temples on the islands of Cos and Delos to enjoy the beauty and silence of the location and to meet with the priests who were acting as dream interpreters, therapists and spiritual guides. The patient stayed at the temple as long as needed for the psyche and the body to be cleansed of its *miasma*. In the Middle Ages, pilgrimages and retreats in monasteries were occasions to break away from family and village, and find solitude, silence and beauty. Later, in the less religious society of nineteen century Europe, the wealthy cured their depressive moods by going to thermal stations in pleasant little cities. With the development of the railways, it became fashionable to leave one's family and spend weeks or months in those luxurious palaces. In France alone, there were hundreds of those Villes D'Eau: Vichy, Evian, Avene, Aix-les-Bains, Contrexeville,Vittel… The patients were expected to bathe in the pools, get a massage everyday, walk, drink lots of the healing local water during the day – and excellent local wines at dinner–, eat good food, go to concerts, dance, make new acquaintances, maybe have romantic or sexual affairs and rest in a quiet hotel room. Today, neuroscience confirms that the inclusion in a non-stressful, pleasant, intellectually or erotically stimulating group is excellent medicine for the depressed brain. Psychologists have long known that libido goes up with the positive contagion of a group that cultivates laughter, deep conversation, friendship and libido goes down with the contagion of a group that breeds competition, stress, anger, fear, and resentment. Recent studies on the phenomenon of the *mirror neuron* explain the neurological basis for that kind of emotional contagion: "because each person continuously emits emotional signals and receives emotional signals that alter him, remarkable things happen when you put people together in a group. Each person's emotional tone is influenced by every other person present. If enough people have a similar emotion, then the positive feedback quickly multiplies so that every person in the group shares a single, intense emotion." [74] The mirror neuron phenomenon is mostly an imitative behavior, which is why neuroscientists often refer to the wider concept *of limbic resonance*, or *limbic regulation*, to point at the wider aspect of our emotional connectedness.

It is important to know that you cannot get uplifting contagion by watching television or playing video games, alone in front of a screen. Virtual relationships severely limit the possibility of *limbic regulation* and only adds to the isolation that is the most common defense mechanism against the hurt of human relations. We like to think that adolescents are the most vulnerable to computer addiction, but there are more and more adults (especially retired adults) whose main occupation is to sit in front of a screen, be it the screen of the television or that of the computer. It occupies the intellect, it kills time, but fails to deliver the benefits that can only come from the physical presence of other beings interacting on an emotional level.

When a long sojourn in a thermal station became fashionable in Europe, other individuals of that same social class went for equally long psychoanalytic treatments in Vienna, with Doctor Freud, or in Zurich with Doctor Jung, or in Paris, London, New York, Boston. While undergoing this *talking cure*, the patients were expected to leave behind, for the duration of the therapy, their professional and familial engagements and free themselves of responsibilities. The typical patient in psychoanalysis, then and there, would often come to reside in the city of the psychoanalyst and would start the day by writing his or her dreams in a diary, to be discussed later with the psychoanalyst, at the rate of three or four sessions a week. This intense introversion was balanced by an active social life, the psychoanalytic community of patients and doctors forming a kind of social club where patients not only discussed their treatment but developed deep friendships and affairs with each others.[75]

Whether you call it retreat, pilgrimage, introversion, incubation, meditation, or the silence of patience, does not matter much. I know a student who found an equivalent by getting in his car and driving from the Atlantic to the Pacific with a stack of CDs', a long meditation on wheels; another found the right atmosphere in walking the seven hundred miles of the Compostelle Way, although he was an atheist; and still another who, through a house exchange network exchanged his house with somebody residing in Toulon, France. To get some company he took classes to become a chef. The point is to find an atmosphere that does not feed the useless fantasy of the Return of Beloved and that offers meditative solitude. Meditation has many similarities with psychotherapy.[76] Although psychotherapy places more emphasis on the *naming* and *analyzing* of emotions, both techniques imply a radical and silent presence to oneself, a quiet acceptance of *what is*. Solitude and introversion are crucial in breaking the fusional state that kept you hooked on incessant, agitated, vapid efforts to reconnect[77].

CHAPTER 7

AH! JEALOUSY

One of the most unpleasant feelings of all is the sense
that somebody is trying to take away our object of love.
No human being can claim to be completely free of
jealousy because it comes with our instinctual territory.
The crocodile says: "This is my lunch and I won't let it
go!" The kitten says: "I'm fighting for the tit because if
I can't get access to it, I'll die." Many a parent has heard
their child declare with the utmost natural: "Mom, let's
return the new baby to the hospital, I really don't want it
here." The child has to be *taught* to tolerate the frustration
of having to share mom's services and understand
instinctively that trashing the new baby may threaten the
essential connection to Mom! Even an only child will
experience jealousy: "If mom has other priorities besides
precious little me, such as sex with Dad, friends she likes
to entertain, the advancement of her career, books she likes
to read… it may signal that I don't count anymore, she
might forget me, I might be abandoned, I'll die." Freud
sexualized rivalry, calling it the oedipal complex ("I wish

143

to kill daddy to have mommy all to myself") but today's neuroscience brings it back to a pre-sexual issue: survival. The word "rival" originally meant two people living on opposite sides of the same river: the word for "bank" in French is "rive." Rivalry is what happens when both sides fight for the same resource: water, milk, food, territory, money, love, sex. Unfair taxation, political injustices, family feuds, all have the same archetypal quality: "Move over so I can access the resource." The expression *the milk of human kindness*, which means compassion, is one of the oldest metaphors equating the breast with everything that one may need in order to survive. Jealousy and rivalry are as ancient as the history of humanity, and as inevitable because of the survival instinct combined with the scarcity of some resources. A rival who takes all the milk from the breast, all the water from the river, all the food from the cellar, all the dollars from the account, all the tax money from the state, threatens the survival of the less powerful ones. Jealousy has been called the oldest sin in the world, because the temptation to eliminate the rival spares no one. Jealousy is first felt as a physical reptilian urge, then it spreads in the limbic brain as a generalized panic. If the education of the young is faulty, or if the code of law is biased against one group or one gender, or if the so called neurons in the "moral brain"[78] have been destroyed, the moral "breaks" are not there to stop jealous acting out. Jealousy then becomes one of the darkest zones of the human heart.

Nietzsche's admiration for the moral genius of the Greeks had to do not only with their recognition of the dark sentiments like jealousy, but with their capacity to upgrade those sentiments into something that has value. Ancient Greek wisdom suggested that the best revenge against jealousy is to do better than the competitor. For example, if the rival community takes an unfair amount of the water, it may propel a community to invent the technique of drilling a well, which eventually gives them better access to water than before. Are we fighting for oil? Let's invent alternative energy sources that will eventually bring more wealth. Are we fighting for territory? Let's explore new territories. Are we fighting for love? Let's multiply the sources of love. Such wisdom elevates the community, making a virtue of a necessity. Many historians have pointed out how issues of fairness in the use of the water in Ancient Mesopotamia was the motivation for the formulation of rules and regulations which evolved into one the most sophisticated code of law that had ever been written; their code of law became a model for all civilizations. Mesopotamia means "the land between the two rivers," which means that people could access to the Tigris-Euphrates river system from four different banks! What was at first a cause for lethal rivalry also created the impetus to evolve. The institution of slavery, as well as the sexual proprietary attitude towards women, have a similar history: the law that forbids your neighbor from diverting the river has the same ultimate goal as the laws that prevent (or should prevent) a master from owning a slave, a husband from killing or maiming his wife because he suspects her (his private property) of infidelity. The objective is to supersede the crocodile, supersede the puppy, and move to a person-to-person relationship as opposed to a person-to-object relationship. Unfortunately, not everyone on this planet has reached that level of moral development, confirming that moral values do follow a process of evolution, just like medical science or technology. The history of our dark sentiments shows how *all* progressive countries moved, or are moving, toward equalitarian laws on two parallel issues; one has to do with collective resources and the need to prevent employers, heads of states, politicians, from behaving as if they owned the people, the land and the resources. Of course, it is an ideal, and we are not always acting according to our values; nonetheless, the moral direction is toward fairness in our code of law and enforcement of order. The other issue where our laws are in constant evolution deals with private behaviors, to prevent husbands and parents from behaving as if they owned their wives and children. Some cultures or nations are more advanced then others in this evolution, a discrepancy that is at the core of the argument in favor of a planetary culture, to preserve collective natural resources, limit procreation and protect the dignity of all human beings.

When a rival deprives us of our object of love, the *feeling* is a murderous one but the *behavior* can be otherwise. A lack of control on one's primitive feelings presents not only a risk of negative legal consequences, but it also harms, what, in us, has the power to set us free. The jealous instinct, like the arousal of primitive anger, leads to a psychic state that depth psychology describes as *psychic inflation*. The word *inflation*, when used in relation to the economy, means an increase of currency or credit, relative to the availability of goods and services, which eventually leads to higher prices and devaluation of that currency. Jung used the notion of inflation to mean "a psychic state characterized by an exaggerated and unreal sense of one's own importance, the cause of which is the identification of the subject with an archetypal image."[79] Jung's definition points at the confusion between the partner (the human, limited, fallible person who died, or who rejected you to go with another) and the archetypal Lover, to whom you attribute (why not, this is inflation after all...) a divine power. The Archetypal Lover has the power of the Great Mother and that of God the Father, the power of creation and of destruction, of reward and punishment. Such inflation is a problem of the ego that always wants to amplify its importance: "I am that Divine Child in need of rescue, the Most Lovable Adult in the Cosmos, the Sweetest Person Ever to Exist, the Absolute Attractor of Love; how dare you reject ME?" An inflated personality is someone who has regular indigestion of capital letters, a psychic ballooning! Any *invasion of unconscious contents* results in a puffing up of the ego and inevitably leads to a devaluation of the currency of love. Those unconscious contents which invade the ego can be summarized in a brief formula: it is *everything you failed to mourn*, starting with the loss (or lack) of the exclusive attention of mommy dearest, daddy dearest and all their surrogates.[80]

This loss, or lack, happened in the past, but you never mourned the loss, so it invades you now. Just like the gambler stays glued to the gaming table, convinced that he will recoup his loss and get lucky again, the jealous maniacal person keeps trying, hoping for partner's return, like a gambler hoping for his luck to turn. Indulging in an addiction always leads to disappointment and failure yet, the addict keeps doing it anyway. Gamblers *know* their addiction threatens their financial security, harms their relationships, destroys their health, but it does not stop them. Jealousy has similar features: it provokes an extravagant expense of psychic energy, with the certainty of failure. In neuroscientific terms jealousy is the result of the billions of synaptic connections that used to bond us first to Mother, then to the partner, and now fail to elicit a reaction, making us as jealous as the five-year-old child who want that new baby to go back where it came from. Neuroscience uses the term "neural memory" while depth psychological uses the term of an *invasion of unconscious contents,* or *unmourned losses.* However one chooses to call it, *it* actually prevents us from experiencing the novelty of an adult relationship between two equal partners, because the brain cannot develop new connections as long as we keep passively waiting for the same stimulation. As Einstein is often quoted to have said: "insanity consists in doing the same thing repeatedly while expecting a different result." Einstein's definition of madness applies as well to obsessive and controlling behaviors stemming from jealousy: it does not inspire Love, and always leads to the moral bankruptcy of the relationship.

There is only one way *around* jealousy. First, you have to *admit* jealousy. Second, as a preventive measure, you should tip-toe away from situations that provoke it. And third, it helps to find pleasure in as many situations as possible. Developing multiple sources of pleasure is like digging a second water well, to end scarcity; it starts with a curiosity for other things and other persons aside from the sexual partner. New sources of pleasure create new pleasurable synaptic associations; it brings your attention away from the situation that provokes jealousy, and it feeds your brain its daily pleasure diet.

For the person mourning a dead partner, jealousy takes the form of a related emotion: envy. Jealousy is a reaction to someone stealing what you feel is yours (your dinner, your money, your partner…) while envy is the disappointment in not having what others have. The widowed are not jealous, but often envious: "Why did I lose my partner to death while they still have theirs?"). The emotion of envy needs to be treated just like that of jealousy: don't beat yourself for feeling it, but move beyond it, otherwise you will never again be able to enjoy your life as it is now.

As humans with a neocortex, we are capable of *taking our distance* from the jealous or envious freak in us, just as we can take our distance from the crocodile and the fearful baby. Our brain can follow the same evolution that produced the advances in our culture. The jealous reflex can never be erased from the brain, no more than the startle reflex; nor can the limbic panic, because we remain vulnerable to loss of love. Nevertheless, just like the building of positive addictions is the most powerful strategy against destructive addictions, another set of reactions can supersede the jealous destructive behaviors. "Ok, I am having a fit of jealousy. I need to make an urgent call to the wise human in me, to prevent jealous acting out."

Moral consciousness, like rationality and scientific empiricism, like our propensity to think philosophically, to imagine artistically, to understand historically, is part of what we are capable of, as human beings. Moral consciousness helps overcome jealousy. Anything that is part of our culture, can be part of your psyche; the richer the culture you insert yourself in, the richer your psyche! Consider this: jealousy is an emotion with a history. The sentiment of jealousy used to be considered absolutely *uncontrollable*, which is why crimes of passion were routinely absolved. Jealousy has evolved into an emotion that is to be expected, but not one a civilized person should *act on*. If *we the people* can evolve by formulating laws that punish crimes of passions like any other crime, so can the individual caught in the jealous emotions brought about by heartbreak. To evolve past your jealous acting out, your brain needs all the help it can get, in order to replace the primitive neural memories of the lost love. That love must be replaced with something *as valuable* as the lost love; you have to move away from pain, toward joy.

CHAPTER 8

TWO FACTORS OF SUSTAINABILITY: JOY AND MEANING

The task of psychotherapy, including self-therapy, is to reestablish lost connections: either the connections between different parts of ourselves –as between the conscious and unconscious– or between ourselves and the world. Traditionally, psychology has interpreted "the world" as meaning "other persons," and consequently has put the emphasis on relationships. It is now becoming evident, through neuroscience, that the psyche is impacted by *everything* in "the world', all animate and inanimate forms in which nature expresses itself. In short, the brain/ psyche is part of an ecological system and like all such systems, its health depends on the *capacity to endure*, which is the definition of sustainability. My understanding of the approach that calls itself eco-psychology, is that all psychology always was, and always will be, an eco-psychology. How can it not be? Adding the prefix *eco* to the noun *psychology* is an interesting strategy to bring back to our attention the fact that the psyche, like a lake, a forest, an ocean, like any ecological system, is healthy when it is open to exchanges, and sick when it becomes a closed system. A sick psyche is a closed system, like a lake infested with algae, because the circulation of water is cut off. A healthy psyche is permeable, mutable, liable to change and exchange, feeding on what supports life, and fading when intoxicated.

A horse won't drink polluted water and will walk long distances to find another water hole, but a closed, sick psyche has lost that instinct, which explains why *giving good advice* inevitably fails with individuals who have gotten more or less adapted to toxic relationships. Their toxic relationships *are* the only family they have, the infested lake they call home. An algae does not have the capacity to move out of the lake, to take residence somewhere else; a human does. But before that person can move away from toxicity, the instinct that prevents the horse from drinking polluted water has to be reactivated. I like to imagine our lifelong quest for wisdom as a continuous process of detoxification, a moving away from situations and relationships that can't support life.

William is a healthy enough person, and the conclusion of his story shows how he was able to *separate*, not so much from Laura, who remained a friend, but from what, in that relationship was unsustainable. We saw how William's awareness of his anger contained the energy to send the final email to Laura, actively breaking the bond. The day after writing his last email to Laura, William went online, and rented a small studio near Kensington Gardens in London. In that really small but quiet apartment he took time to rest, read, discover the city, and work on his dissertation for his second Ph.D. It also gave him some peace and quiet that the heart needs to heal. At the end of July, after a month of solitude, he felt ready for company. He left the tiny flat in London and rented a summer house in Ireland. The house had three bedrooms and was near the coast. He invited his daughters, their friends, and two of his old friends from the university to come visit. He sent me the following email:

I READ, I WALK, I SWIM, I SLEEP, I HEAL.

I read novels, I walk the cliffs with my friends, I swim with my daughters, I sleep long nights, I drink lots of tea, I cook big meals and I like how the world feels, with or without Laura in it. I am on a treasure hunt in search of my lost self. I congratulate myself every day on the fact that I have stopped spending my days and sleepless nights waiting, hoping for Laura to change her mind and to choose me over Jack. I still miss her affection, her caresses, her presence but it is now a quiet kind of sadness that does not prevent me from enjoying the beauty of the place, here, and the presence of friends and family.

Laura's betrayal reduced me to a pathetic helpless beggar and I see that she had that power over me because of the unconsciousness of my history with my mom. My mother made me beg for her love, as if I was never quite good enough to be worthy of it. Laura triggered that reaction in me. Of course, it is not just my "mother complex": there is the real, actual loss of Laura, which is not part of my past, it is happening now. Yet, the more I become aware of the unconscious mother-wound, the more I see its immense influence on my relationships to all the women in my life, and not only with Laura. I still feel vulnerable, as if my heart had been forced open and I am not yet competent at protecting it.

I am not angry at Laura anymore, I understand her. Two worlds collided. Laura's world is a constant doing, in survival mode, with urgent goals and ambitions. She has more challenges then she can meet in a day because she is still creating her vocation, finding her way in the world. My goal is very different probably because I am older and more secure professionally. I want my life to contain more peace, more joy, more pleasure, away from goal setting. Sooner or later our incompatible world views would have broken our relationship.

I am at peace with myself and with Laura.

By spending three months in Europe, William was literally forcing his brain to learn an unfamiliar surrounding and he was creating new sources of pleasure and joy.

It is never enough to express the *intention* of letting go, not enough to state: "It's over, I am letting go of you." One has to *activate* that choice by doing enough concrete changes for the brain to register that the situation is new and can be pleasurable if one can adapt to the novelty. Like animals undergoing a major climate change, or a population of humans during a war, a devastating epidemic, a revolution, the brain gets busy creating many new synaptic connections. That neuronal activity is the best medicine for heartbreak, because the brain *gets it* that the attachment to the partner is not serving life anymore. Letting go does *not* mean one becomes indifferent to the person that was once loved, but rather *that the addiction is separated from the affection.* If the relationship has enough gold in it; in other words, if there is true love, it will find its proper form, later.

A heartbroken friend of mine did a wine tour of the Napa Valley with a group of French wine enthusiasts; another, who was a school psychologist, started to pay attention to all the adolescents in his school who were suffering from heartbreaks; he designed a program to help them. That project helped him as much as it helped them. Over the years, I have heard from many of my adult students that writing their dissertation was their way of resurfacing from a heartbreak, or from a loss, or a failed enterprise. Studying occupies the mind, which give the heart a break, while one forges a new identity. Institutions of higher learning, especially those where the students form a cohesive group, –like the one at which I teach[81] – offer the optimal conditions for neurogenesis: a constant flow of new ideas, the familiarity of a group with which to have rich conversations, balanced with long periods of introverted solitude, to do the reading and the writing. These are ideal conditions, as potent as the ancient healing sanctuaries, which is the reason why I chose to stay in a small, not widely known Institute, where teachers love to teach and students love to learn. I appreciate the smallness of it. There is a multitude of ways to create similar conditions, and there are many places that offer those favorable conditions for neurogenesis to happen. It happens only when one is engaged on all fronts: intellectually, emotionally, physically, and socially. This ideal used to be part of the mission of every university, where vast beautiful gardens were meant for conversations and solitary walks, and faculty were passionate about educating the mind and soul of their students. Unfortunately, many of our best and largest institutions of higher learning are often forced to adjust to the dominant values: competition for grants, star status for their professors and international ranking which determines the market value of their diplomas. In pursuit of such goals, the right hemisphere of the brain often fails to get its daily diet of meaning and joy.

Most theories about psychological healing agree that renewal comes with *psychic movement*; something, however small, starts to *move* in the psyche –a new metaphor for an old tired situation, a different feeling about something, a sudden curiosity – and the psyche starts coming out of its torpor. This movement may be a tiny psychic move, but as the momentum grows, it gets you out of bed, out of the house, out of the emotional prison of heartbreak. Reciprocally, physical sluggishness brings psychological stagnation because the outer and the inner are connected. True movement is not an *agitation,* not a stirring of the same contaminated brew. You can recognize a real move of the psyche, as opposed to agitation, by the fact that what has been hurting in the recent past, shows signs of abating; neurogenesis is pulling the psyche in the new direction. A real *move* permeates life with a sense of adventure.

William had been subjected to mild neglect and coldness from his mother; his family history contained no episodes of physical abuse, no stories of addictions, violence, or dangerous neglect. The task of re-establishing sustainability in a very abused (polluted) psyche is evidently more arduous, although not necessarily more painful than it was for William. The next vignette tells the story of a man who realized that the task of helping his wife become a happier person was beyond his capacity. Edward realized that his wife Elise couldn't or wouldn't separate from her toxic family, psychically imprisoned in a closed system that was not life-sustaining. There was no room to include him, the outsider who was suggesting to his wife to leave the infested location! His instincts told him to take his distance. Like a healthy horse, Edward walked away to find another water source.

THE POLLUTED FISHBOWL

Elise would tell me every day that she loved me; she cajoled and kissed and sweet talked me. At the beginning of our marriage, three years ago, I asked her to reserve her vacation time to travel with me in Italy. Traveling is my most intense source of pleasure; I want to see as much as I can of this beautiful world before I am too old to travel. I am interested in other cultures, other climates, traveling is my main motivation to make money. Elise always said she would travel with me, but when the time came to buy our tickets, she said she couldn't because she needed to visit her mother in Tuscaloosa, Alabama. Her mother, according to Elise, was having a very difficult time with her health, and was under great stress because of the drama of the divorce of her other daughter (Elise's sister). The same thing happened again the second year of our marriage, and again this Spring. Last week, she informed that her Summer vacation will again be spent in Tuscaloosa, not Tuscany.

Elise's mother has endless claims on Elise's free time, money, vacation time, attention and emotions; Elise does not have the strength to put any kind of limit. Her mom calls every day, sometimes twice a day and with all kinds of demands. Elise is not free to be my partner, not open to anything but the influence of her sanctimonious, controlling, invasive, egocentric mother.

*I understand and appreciate Elise's desire to help
her family, and I would contribute, if not for the fact
that I feel Elise's efforts are futile because her mom,
as well as her sister, appears to me as vampiristic
takers. These two woman have denied themselves so
much, they will take and take and take from Elise and
still won't give her the love and respect she craves.
Elise's mother expects her daughter to serve her like
the queen bee, to sacrifice her (our) vacation time year
after year; I am never part of their equation, nor is
Elise right to happiness and calm.*

*My irreversible disconnection from Elise happened
over something that may seem like a detail. We were
listening to a new CD I had bought that afternoon and
I was looking forward to a pleasant evening of music.
Just as we settled down to listen, her mother called on
the phone, with another episode of her ongoing drama.
Elise listened to her mother's litany of complaints for
an hour. After ten minutes of waiting, I had lost the
desire to listen to the music and felt a huge let down. I
had a sudden certitude: Elise is incapable of grasping
the meaning of "us," the importance of our vacation
time, of our evenings. Her psyche lives in a polluted
fishbowl, with her neurotic mom and her neurotic
sister. I will suffocate if I stay. I left the CD on the
table, went out for a walk, and knew, there and then,
that I had to ask for a divorce.*

Edward used his judgment to end a relationship that was not sustainable because Elise was still trying to please her mother, who just can't be pleased! We first learn to succeed and to fail in our family: "Look Dad! Am I worthy of your love? Not yet? Let me try harder... here, is this enough?... not quite ?... but look at this success, isn't it real?" In a healthy enough family, when a child finally leaves behind the dependency of adolescence and becomes an independent adult, with both a capacity to love and to earn a living, the parents are grateful, and they bless their child as he/she leaves the nest. The young healthy adult is happy to find work, which allows independence and gives something back to society, in exchange for the education he/she received. In a neurotic family, like Elise's, the mother herself has remained immature. She never reached the level of psychic autonomy that would allow her to let go of her daughters; they are in service to their mother's needy psyche and it suffocates the whole family.

Nature teaches *avoidance* as much as it teaches *connection*. Mammals learn what food they can eat, and what food is poisonous; they learn to bond and they learn to avoid predators. A healthy psyche learns the same: avoid individuals who oppress and abuse, and connect with those who liberate and sustain. In a relationship, when no amount of giving and loving is ever enough to fill the void, it is better to sidestep, let go, move out and find another niche. Elise's mother had an abysmally polluted psyche, but Elise's instincts were distorted; like a horse who can't smell the pollution, she kept drinking from the contaminated well. There is not much Edward could do to help her. Psychotherapists also have that kind of experience, with patients whose goal in therapy is to confirm that nobody has the power to help them.

Eco-psychology

Humans are joy-seekers, and meaning-seekers; both joy and meaning are the foundations on which rest our system of values. If we are coherent, our values determine our behaviors, in other words, we walk the talk. A child is born, and suddenly we feel how *joyful* and *meaningful* it is to keep that baby alive, joining the vast community of humans who found it joyful and meaningful to do so, since the beginning of humanity. The joy and meaning of keeping a baby alive reveals the *value* we give to human life, and to the continuity between the generations. In turn, the *value* determines the *behavior*: we'll feed, protect, educate the little ones, even if it deprives us of sleep, costs a fortune and takes an exorbitant amount of emotional energy. Abusive parents typically did not have a *joyful* nor a *meaningful* experience at the birth of their child: it just happened because they had sex. They may give lip service to the *value* of that child but really, there is a discrepancy between the value they profess and their behavior. Growing up in a house were there are few occasions of joy creates a profound unbalance between the forces of life and the forces of death. Sooner or later that unbalance becomes unsustainable for the psyche. It can be corrected if joy is introduced anew in adult life, and fresh meaning discovered. The existentialist philosopher Jean

Paul Sartre once remarked that suffering seems to contain more *being* than the positive emotions of joy and love. He calls that a *cultural bewitchment*. Painful emotions do seem truer, says Sartre, only because our Christian religious values have taught us to respect sacrifice and pain, more than they taught us respect for joy and pleasure. Sartre's philosophical insight finds a validation in the language of neuroscience: a rigid and dogmatic culture, whose values are sacrificial, oppressive and violent, molds our brain circuitry in such a way that pain, sacrifice and frustration, come to have more neuronal connections than play, delight, curiosity, joy.

Meaning follows *value*, even if the value comes vicariously, obliquely. What is the *meaning* of a garden? Difficult to say! Flowers don't add proteins to your diet, they need care, space, and they cost money. Add the "ing" that transforms the noun into the verb, and one finds that *gardening* has been a meaningful activity for kings and queens, for the rich and for the poor, for the amateurs and the professionals. In absolutely all great cultures, the art of gardening is valued. Anybody who likes gardening can testify it can give meaning and joy. One can also discover where meaning is located, via a failure to act; stop caring for your garden and see how you feel. Stop caring for you house and feel how depressing a slovenly house can be, revealing the value of good housekeeping. Stop caring for your pet and see how you feel when it dies. The meaning of any given experience is not always as obvious as keeping our baby alive and the house in good repair. In relationships, meaning is also revealed by the way one walks the talk, even in small matters of domestic partnership. Words are expected to *mean* something, and the words "I love you" are definitely one of our biggest statement, but it can mean all or nothing.

The next vignette is about a young man of thirty-two, whose girlfriend, Cindy, wastes joy, like others waste money, as if joy was not a most precious ingredient to sustain psychic life. When he abruptly terminated their relationship, it was a devastating shock to her, because she had never learned to consider how little things can carry big meaning and joy.

CINDY'S PROMISES

On my first birthday we celebrated together, Cindy asked what would please me. I suggested taking singing lessons together, because I love to sing with her. She promised she would call a voice teacher she knows, but then she forgot. I reminded her a few weeks later, and she said: "My workload is intense. Let's postpone the singing lessons until the Summer." Summer arrived and I reminded her again. She said: "Oh, yes, yes. Sure. I am going to take care of it." She forgot. A year later, again for my birthday, she asked me what I would like for a gift. "Singing lessons with you" I replied. Months went by, but still nothing. Then I thought that maybe singing lessons might not be such a great idea for us, because it didn't seem to appeal to her, otherwise she would have kept her promise. And I thought that maybe the problem was that I wasn't assertive enough. So, I let go of the idea of singing lessons, and formulated a different and very clear demand: "This Sunday, I would like us to go hiking, with our backpacks and a picnic, and swim with you in the creek that runs beside the trail." That was a clear enough program! "Fantastic," she said. Sunday morning comes, but then her girlfriend calls and asks Cindy to come help her finish the painting job of her dining room, because she has guests coming the next day and she can't have them come with a half finished job. The friend is asking two hours of Cindy's time, but it turns out it takes the whole Sunday and I spend it alone. It may look like a tiny incident, but when I brought it up, Cindy lectured me on the importance of friendship, and blah blah blah. I suddenly realized that her values about what constitutes a good life are absolutely incompatible with mine. She is not someone who has talent for happiness; she spoils every occasion with unnecessary complications. She has that same avarice when it comes to giving us sexual time. The truth is that she never defends our pleasures; there is always something else she wants to do. I don't like our life together.

Cindy *said* she loved her partner, yet she repeatedly forgot to *act* on those words. The promise of singing lessons may seem trivial, but had she been attentive to her partner, she would have known that for him, singing *meant* joy. She repeatedly destroyed his joy until he could not trust any of her words of love.

Neurotically handicapped individuals have learned a parasitic form of survival: they plug themselves on the power source of another being, and no amount of nurturing will convince them to unplug. If you have ever ridden on a tandem bicycle with somebody who only goes through the motions of moving their legs up an down, without applying any muscular energy, you know what a parasitic relationship feels like. As long as you contribute the muscle power to move the wheels, it works. You stop? The motion stops. You start again? The partner is willing to go along, as long as you provide the propulsion energy. These individuals don't seem to know that the partner can *feel* their laziness. Theirs is mock energy, fake participation, vampiristic sucking. The rational solution is to stay away from such parasitic individuals, but if you have the matching neurosis– which is a poor sense of self-worth– you will be attracted to them!

The balanced human

The malleability of our brain explains why, in the long history of humanity, there are two variables that seem to predict the resilience of any given culture: the first one is the capacity of a people to develop left brain rational solutions to practical problems: science and technology. Cholera epidemics, that were historically responsible for the death of millions, are a good example of what happens when there is no rational understanding of the causes of the disease and a lack of medical technology for such an easily treatable disease. The second variable is the level of *creativity* (right brain) in bringing forth new values, via the arts and the humanities (for example values that promote hygiene and education). Those two variables explain why every successful culture has given importance to the development of *both* science and the humanities. This need for an equilibrium finds a parallel in the process of overcoming heartbreak: you need to understand *why* your brain reacts with such intensity to a heartbreak. The examination of causal links belongs to the scientific method and it is important to look at your heartbreak as you would look at any other health problem. But that is not all: you also need a creative, inventive, imaginative response to modify the *symbolic milieu* in which you will either thrive or fail to thrive. As Allan Guggenbuhl writes: "The love experience cannot be comprehended adequately in relational terms and it does not originate in causes. The partners realize that something more, something inexplicable is happening to them. Soul has chosen the encounter between two people to express its power and energy."[82] That something more and inexplicable is the resonance from the unconscious, which emerges in symbolic form.

A rich culture is not formulaic, not simplistic, not superstitious, not inflated; it teaches its youth to think rationally *and* it tries to communicate the wisdom accumulated in the humanities. The humanities are the voice that says to expect light and shadow, pain and joy. In a rich culture, scientists are responsible for technological progress and medical advances, while artists symbolize and express our changing values to give meaning to our shared humanity. Similarly, your psyche needs that kind of richness to relate to the wise person in your brain.

CHAPTER 9

REAL LOVE AND FALSE LOVE: THE CHANCES OF GETTING BACK TOGETHER

Don't go away, Don't go away. [...] I will sing about those great lovers who saw both their hearts flower anew. [...] Fiery flames can arise from a volcano that was thought extinct...Don't go away, Don't go away...

Lyrics of "Ne Me Quitte Pas."
Jacques Brel

We all know of couples who split apart only to discover that the suffering that separated them has also created the conditions for a renewal; they get back together after a hiatus and continue to evolve as a couple. Stories of reunion are inspiring, but they are also dangerous; they can keep us hooked on hope, hope for the wrong thing! When love is *real*, it doesn't just fade away like a skin rash; it may resurface after an eclipse. Yet, for psychology to be able to define *real love* would first require a stable definition of what is *real* and not real *in the psychic realm*, a distinction that is impossible to make because the psyche evolves as the culture evolves. Secondly, it would require a stable definition of *love* – how many parts of neurotic dependency for how many parts of healthy attachment. Psychology has none of those stable definitions!

Psychology came out of the medical model, concerned with the treatment of the sick psyche, which always was and still is much easier to define than the normal psyche. The instrument of our profession, the Diagnosis Statistical Manual (DSM), now in preparation for its fifth edition, offers precise and empirical definitions of all kinds of pathologies, but none of normalcy; again, because our definition of normalcy evolves with the culture. The list of what is in or out of the DSM is a very unstable one; homosexuality was previously perceived as a sickness, now it isn't. The next version (DSM 5, due in 2013) is expected to include a few new categories, among which a development of the notion of the Passive–Aggressive Personality as a behavior that "manifest a learned helplessness, procrastination, stubbornness, resentment, sullenness, or deliberate/repeated failure to accomplish requested tasks for which one is (often explicitly) responsible"[83].

The actual DSM IV presently offers a comprehensive analysis of the many aspects of the love addiction, under many rubrics, yet the DSM never had anything to say about the meaning and mystery of *real* love. In lieu of stable definitions for love we find in the humanities a richness of *symbols* and stories, to express what humans understand as *real love*. The most stable and universal symbol for it has always been gold because it remains untarnished by the passage of time; it doesn't waste even in the most corrosive conditions; it radiates light and warmth; it is a beautiful metal. Likewise, "real love" won't tarnish even in adverse conditions (infidelity, betrayal, separation, old age and sickness.)[84]

The ancient art of alchemy, with its catalogue of metaphors to choose from, is an example of the historical need for a rich repertoire of symbols to symbolize the transformative power of *real* love. For the alchemists, the metal lead was a symbol of depression and gloom; yet lead could be transformed into gold. If you compare lead with neurotic attitudes, and real love with gold, you can appreciate the whole deep symbolism of the processes *of alchemical transmutation*.[85] In any new relationship, love sparkles and shines because it is untested. If the alloy (the relationship) is rich enough in gold, it will sustain the acid of time. The overcoming of difficulties will purify love of its infantile attachments, and *transmute* the sexual urge into the golden sentiment of love. Old couples who have loved each other over a lifetime, at the moment of the ultimate separation of death, often express that, at the end, only the gold remains; gone are the resentments, reproaches, grievances, all has been purified. It is indeed a beautiful paradox that a great love makes the final farewell more bearable. Knowing that one has loved, and has been loved, is a reward of a life well lived, the real gold, the alchemical *opus*.

If there is such a thing as *real love*, it implies there is also *false love*: as soon as the thin romantic plating wears down, the relationship become leaden. Lead, considered by the alchemists as a base metal, is as old a symbol as gold, to symbolize a kind of heaviness and lack of luster that is contrary to love. Another metaphor for false love is that of *fool's gold*, (iron pyrite) which only looks like gold but is not. It was used by the alchemists to create "oil of vitriol" (sulfuric acid). Fool's gold, is not only an acute disappointment for the literal gold digger, it is also a substance that, when oxidized, becomes explosive[86]. In the psychological realm, a relationship that is mostly in the service of neurotic defenses is fool's gold. In such cases, divorce is always better than trying to work on the relationship. Deciding which is which (real gold or fool's gold) can be helped by examining how the relationship either liberates or imprisons.

The younger we are, the more our relationships are burdened with projections, because of the need to repair the still fresh wounding of having gone through childhood and adolescence. It is quite natural for young lovers to confuse *declarations* of love with love, because *the imagination of love* must compensate for a reality that has yet to be created. It is only when the sweet words of the honeymoon bump against the harsh reality of coupledom that the golden plating starts to wear out.

Past the time of romantic infatuation, individuals who create or remain in leaden relationships usually do so because that is how they have *learned* to relate. For them, gloom, boredom, oppression, confusion, frigidity, humiliation, retaliation... all feel completely *natural*. They take turns manipulating each other in order to remain in the well charted territory of their complementary neurosis. Both sides may suspect that they may be missing something about the glory of love, but they can't quite put words on it. A couple's neurotic structure can fit like puzzle pieces, giving a false sense of belonging. I remember a young patient, Monica, who complained a lot about her young husband: "He is cold and detached and unconnected." She could have added "Just like my father," but she did not see that connection, nor could she see how willingly she cast herself in the corresponding role of domestic and sexual commodity. She bitterly resented her financial dependency, and lashed at her husband with incessant financial recriminations, but did nothing to emancipate herself, she did not seem interested in getting a training and a job. She expected no pleasure out of their sexual life, and gave little in return. This frigidity, this loneliness, this boredom *felt natural* to her. As for her husband, whom I also met, he felt that love was the most overrated sentiment of all times, and sexuality not much more than relief of an itch. What brought them to therapy is a recommendation from their family doctor, who insisted that they do a few sessions in couple therapy, before prescribing yet another anti-depressant for her, and yet another anxiolytic drug for him. It did not take long to conclude that they both wanted, and needed, a divorce. She continued therapy; a year later she formulated the psychological insight that led her away from that loveless relationship.

I HAD NO MODEL FOR A LOVING RELATIONSHIP

As an adolescent, I understood that my father had no interest whatsoever in raising a daughter, dismissing me as if my very existence was a bad trick destiny played on him. As a rebellion, I married someone who, at first, seemed pleased with my "services" and valued my domestic capacity; I believed that being a good servant to his needs would save me from feeling like trash. I soon reproduced, with my husband, the same situation as with my father, it felt like the only option. My husband had been as unloved as I had; his mother was weak and self-centered; she expected him, the son, to take the responsibilities his father did not want to carry. He chose a wife like myself, who detested herself, and who wanted to remain financially dependent on him. As an adolescent, my husband took on the role of provider to an unhappy mother and since this was the only model of relating he had learned, he defended himself by developing aloofness and detachment. He worked too much, drank too much, ate too much, and neither he nor I could understand what was missing. We had no models, no symbols, no stories about the kind of playful generosity that naturally flows from love. Our restricted relationship felt slightly better than what we had experienced in our families: my husband was a relatively stable provider, an improvement on my irresponsible father. As for my husband, he had more ways of avoiding me, his wife, than he had had of avoiding his parasitic mother; having me as a wife felt like an improvement on his adolescence. Both of us yearned for something unknown.

In my experience, that kind of leaden marriage is best terminated by divorce, because none of the partners can teach the other the alchemical art of transmuting lead into gold. Her divorce forced Monica to move to the city, go back to school and train as a nurse. She found a community of friends, where she learned new patterns of being and the meaning of the word *joy*. Her training, and her new network of friends compensated for her delayed maturation. As for her husband, the month after their divorce, he had a sexually hot affair with an uninhibited and very loveable woman, and for the first time in his life, he felt that *making love* could actually *produce* love! This experience did to him what a climate change does to some species of animals: a boost in evolution. For both of them, married life had been a regressive leaden state; there had been so little gold in their union that marriage used it all up. Their divorce was a positive move, helping both of them dissolve the paralyzing parental projections. Their relationship was not abusive in the legal sense of domestic abuse, yet, it was robbing both of them of the possibility of golden moments.

The distinction between a relationship which is *difficult* but also contains much gold, and one that is difficult because it is abusive (one which contains mostly lead) is not easy to establish, but it is well worth the effort. Helping our partner through rough times is a mark of love, but helping someone incapable or unwilling to reciprocate always reveals a neurotic collusion, turning the nurturer into what in AA is called an "enabler." Psychologically healthy individuals have their own power source, and they replenish themselves by the air they breathe, the food their eat, the work they do, the rest they take, the love they get *and the love they give*.

The next chapter examines another dark corner of the human soul, one that asks for a lot of weeding and clearing out of the debris to see the sun.

CHAPTER 10

NARCISSISM AND GRIEF

The breakup of an intimate relationship is a huge narcissistic wound, maybe the most acute. Typically, both partners will feel that *the other* is the one showing self-centeredness and narcissistic selfishness: "After all I did for you…the least you could do… " feels the abandonee. "Give me a break, I want out, I have given you enough, this time it's about me, not about you" may feel the abandoner.

Issues of narcissism –our own as well as our partner's– are a crucial aspect of the process of rehabilitation. Narcissism tends to limit to a purely utilitarian nature, the exchanges one has with the world, as well as with others. We easily accept that a burn victim experiencing severe pain will be concerned mainly with his/her own suffering; the professional caretakers don't expect otherwise, yet our patience with the egocentricity of the sick may wear out. Narcissism does to the psyche what a monoculture (the monoculture of me, me and more me….) does to the environment: an impoverishment that can lead to absolute devastation. The tradition at a wake is to bring food, support, attention, affection to the bereaved, because their loss is so tragic that the whole community is willing to give the bereaved exclusive attention; their pain and their loss is all that counts for a while. Yet, if the widow or widower remains, year after year, in the sad and egocentric emotions brought about by the loss, there is the risk of suffering another loss: the connection to the community. The others feel as if the mourner is saying: "Only my suffering counts, yours is nothing compared to mine." If this attitude persists and define all forms of relationships, it may indicate what psychiatry calls a "Narcissistic Personality Disorder" which describes somebody who is narcissistic all the time, with everybody. We shall see later, with Susan's example, the nine characteristic from the DSM that defines this disorder. For now, enough is to say that a heartbreak brings about many traits of that clinical portrait; after all, you are a mourner. First there is that *"grandiose sense of self-importance"* because you feel as if your loss is like no one else's, more profound, more painful, special, unique, exceptional. Second there is that *"lack of empathy"* for others because you are totally absorbed in yourself and cannot hear nor see others. And most of all there is that narcissistic sense of *"entitlement"* which is so typical of the regressive pull of heartbreak; you feel as if the partner *owes* you love.

The question of narcissism is crucial for another reason: there are two persons involved in a breakup, and two narcissisms clashing. If your partner was a pathological narcissist, the question is: why did you stay in such a partnership? If your partner was not a pathological narcissist, but rather a generous and healthy person, how will you treat your own narcissistic wound? If you don't, you are condemning yourself to isolation and desolation.

If your partner was a narcissist...

It may seem very easy to break-up from a relationship with a selfish, self serving, egocentric, navel-gazer-egomaniac-taker, yet, many decent individuals get caught in their net, and for many reasons. Narcissists can be very seductive, seemingly warm, receptive, and generous, especially in the beginning of a relationship, or in a public context. A narcissist might be rich and famous, and the attention of such a social star might feed your own narcissistic traits. The hook is always our own narcissism, and the narcissist's most clever trick is to use your narcissism as a bait to trap you in a one-way partnership. The fact that narcissism is culturally so well tolerated, does not help us to recognize the type, especially in milieus where success and star status is the main value. Narcissistic parents tend to transmit their narcissistic traits to their kids, which means that as long as the family has the means to maintain a position of social dominance, the parents and their kids can be as narcissistic as they please, and nobody will object. Their failure to love is not perceived because love is a private emotion, its absence not obvious to the Jones, nor to the media.

There are now two major theories about narcissism, one from psychoanalysis and the other from social psychology. They contradict each other, yet, I believe they are both to be considered when deciding which form of narcissism one is dealing with. The first theory is the classical psychoanalytic perspective, when Freud suggested an important distinction between the so called *primary narcissism* which is the normal self-centeredness of the child, as opposed to *secondary narcissism*, which today would be called a healthy self-esteem. Both these forms of narcissism are part of human nature: primary narcissism is to be expected in all kids, while paying attention to the kind of haircut that fits you best, would be an example of secondary narcissism, also a natural and good thing. In Freud's view, when the primary narcissism persists beyond adolescence, it becomes a failure to understand the give-and-take principle of adult human exchange; it becomes a failure of love. In the generations of Freudian followers, a plethora of psychoanalysts (Kohut[87], Horney[88], Masterson[89], Milton,[90]) theorized pathological narcissism as the result of *self-loathing*. The narcissistic personality, in their view, is a defense mechanism against a narcissistic wounding in childhood. In other words, the narcissist inflates his/her value as compensation for feeling so small and worthless: "I make myself so big because I feel so small."

There is another, more recent and contradictory portrait of the narcissist, which is in direct opposition to that *self-loathing individual*. The new theory about narcissism comes from research in social psychology, and offers a very different portrait of the narcissist, as a truly *self-adoring individual*.[91] I think both these perspectives are relevant, because there is more than one brand of narcissism, a voracious plant that spreads like weeds and can grow on both a psychoanalytic or a sociological ground.

If you are recovering from breaking up with a narcissist, it is useful to examine those two theories in detail, and see which one fits your ex-partner, in order to remove the hook that attracted you to such a taker.

The narcissist as a self-loathing individual

Psychoanalytic theory first reversed many of the nineteenth century perceptions, in stating that a narcissist is *not* someone who loves himself/herself; it is someone who *does not know love*; neither love of Self, nor love of Other. A narcissist is cold to himself/herself, as well as to the partner, because he/she is still caught in the infantile rage against the parent, whose approval and support was so needed, yet withheld. It is an individual incapable of *giving* – "I did not get what I needed, why should you?" If there was a bumper sticker to summarize the psychoanalytic theory about narcissism it might read: "I am a narcissist: my curse is a hatred of what I most need –you."

Heinz Kohut's book *The Analysis of the self: A Systematic Analysis of the Treatment of the Narcissistic Personality Disorders,* had a most significant impact in psychiatry, because his definition of the narcissistic personality disorder found its way into the DSM. To become healthy adults, Kohut theorized that children needed to be "mirrored" positively by an "empathically resonant self-object" – by which he meant a family in which you feel valued, with competent adults who can be role models. If not properly *mirrored*, you can catch a narcissistic personality disorder. The cure, according to Kohut, is to find a therapist who can take the place of the parent and, through transference, re-parent the patient. As the patient experiences a "secure attachment" with the therapist, by repeated experience of being "mirrored," –seen, valued– he/she develops a coherent personality structure. Kohut imagines the ideal parent/therapist as someone who responds to the needs of the child/patient with a "non-hostile firmness" and a "non-seductive affection." His insistence on the importance of *empathy* in therapy, was a needed departure from the authoritarian interpretive Freudian frame of reference. Kohut was born in Vienna in 1913, wrote his major work from the fifties to the seventies, and although he did witness the growth of cultural narcissism, his focus was not to address the problem of the generalized "seductiveness" of consumerism, nor to comment on the actual dismal failure to provide a "non-hostile firmness" in education.

Kohut's theory dominated the field of psychoanalytic studies for a generation, although there were some sharp critics. One such critic is that of James Hillman, who sees Kohut's approach to narcissism as a trap for patients: "I keep a distance from the Kohut craze. Although recognizing narcissism as the syndrome of the times [...] Kohut attempts its cure by the same means of narcissistic obsession: an ever more detailed observation of subjectivity. And a subjectivity within the oppressive confines of a negatively reconstructed childhood." [92] In other words, Hillman sees the risk of such an approach in the fact that patients may become ever more fascinated by the story of their trauma, giving less and less attention to others and to the world, always in search of somebody to *mirror* them.

The narcissist as a self-adoring individual

Starting with Christopher Lasch, with his book on *The Culture of Narcissism* (1979), the narcissist was presented not as a victim of poor parenting and wounded self-image, but the result of a culture that breeds narcissism like a cultural virus. The idea that narcissism might be a cultural problem now has the support of research in social psychology, with convincing evidence that the narcissist can be somebody truly *in love with himself* and *only* himself, a going back to the nineteenth century sense, although from a very different approach.

The new theory about narcissism comprises a cultural critique of parents raising children like royalty ("What would you like to be served for dinner, honey?") and it comprises a critique of the economy, which offers credit cards to teenagers and to parents who themselves can't control their spending[93]. That brand of narcissism, characterized by a lack of self-control, is theorized as the result of parents and educators who wrongly believed that giving accolades *raises self-esteem* and *leads to success,* when research proves that it doesn't; in fact it seems to be quite the opposite. Summarizing years of research, by themselves and other social psychologists, Twenge and Campbell[94] describe the narcissist as: 1) somebody who really loves him/her/self first (self-adoration, really); 2) feels entitled way beyond his/her competence; 3) is a handicap for business, because he/she is not a good team worker; 4) hurt those who commit themselves to him/her because he/she will use and abuse friends, co-workers, and spouses; 5) and, finally, he/she becomes a pathetic isolated loser when he/she loses his good looks, or money, or power position.

Narcissism is seen as the natural outcome of a consumerist culture that disconnects freedom from responsibility. Immature parents let their kids get away with irresponsibility because they neurotically *need to be needed,* and to feel approved and loved by their kids, a reversal of the past ideal of children striving for their parent's love and approval.

If you broke up from a relationship with a narcissist, there is no way to decide for sure which of these two contradictory theories applied to your former narcissistic partner. To add to the confusion, there are many self-help books about relationships that carry a heavy load of sentimentality and teach love as universal remedy: ("Show empathy, forget your grudges") while others insist on the opposite ("Show tough love, don't be an enabler"). Which is which?

I believe the solution is to look at arguments from all sides, and decide by yourself if you were dealing with a *self-loathing* narcissist, or with *a self-adoring* narcissist. In the former case you may have discovered, in your partner, an inner voice that whispers: "Anyone who *wants* to be with me must not be worth loving." The problem it creates for you, is that your partner's hungry bottomless wounded ego will gobble every drop of emotional honey you can produce, but that supply will, at the same time, be devalued as worthless. The price to pay is emotional exhaustion and the feeling that you are invisible.

If your partner was a self adoring narcissist, you may have already discovered the unsustainability of being partnered with an immature selfish taker, who wants *you* to be the empathic, nurturing, giving, supportive parent, while he/she remains the spoiled, irresponsible teen, with the credit card and no responsibilities. Can such a partner grow-up? How much are you ready to bet on it?

There is no substitute for developing a good nose, to smell the rats who disguise themselves as Prince Charming, or to detect the Barbies/ Bimbos/ Inflatable Expensive Flesh and Blood Dolls who present themselves as Love Goddesses. At the beginning of your relationship there might have been a period where you felt courted with extraordinary dedication, because he/she offered a kind of attention modeled on his/her own immature ideal of love: romance, gifts, glitter, ego flattering adulation. Gradually, so gradually you may not have seen it, the wooing turned into a grand existential theft, as the partner performed a greedy appropriation of everything in your personality that could serve his/her needs. You discovered a hidden agenda, as if you had signed the following contract: "I will let you use all my talents, feed on my heart, and if my contribution doesn't make your star brighter, or doesn't serve your needs, I agree to be devalued, put down, and discarded as worthless." Your self-adoring partner, stuck in the infantile position of wanting much while contributing little, assigned to you the parental role of caretaker, but with *no reciprocity*. No therapist in the world can tell you for sure if generosity and devotion can ever transform such a partner into someone capable of returning love. The self-adoring narcissist has not yet *learned* to love, and he/she may *not be interested* in learning a non-utilitarian relationship. "Don't bother me, and take care of all the problems" is the basic tune. If your partner is the self-adoring narcissist described by recent research in social psychology, your generosity may end up confirming his/her sense of entitlement. Any adult who is an eternal adolescent, will use you, and your resources, until you have an empty breast, an empty bank account, an empty heart, a dried up soul. Don't try solicitude, patience and support; don't even try "tough love," since it is still a taking on the responsibility of *educating* the partner, like a therapist or a parent can do. In an unsustainable relationship, the wisest thing most healthy people do, is to kick him/her out, disappear from that social circle, cut the money line, make yourself unavailable, detach and leave.

Both approaches, either from psychoanalysis or from social psychology, converge in the admission that narcissism is one of the most difficult problem to tackle and one with cultural dimensions that cannot be ignored. Love exists only between equals, but for narcissists, this notion of equality remains mysterious and illusory. When a narcissist is in the presence of authentic love between two people, he/she cannot grasp it. Narcissists cannot find love because they don't know what they are looking for. They have learned that being loved is equivalent to being "serviced," like a car in a garage, a man at a bordello, a client on the massage table, a patient at the therapist, a customer at the restaurant. The cultural virus that rewards narcissism, has created hordes of people with bottomless needs and vampiristic psyches, a sociological phenomenon that may explain this generation's fascination with vampire stories.

I know of only one person, in my whole career as a psychologist, who successfully tackled her narcissism. I met Susan as an adult student of psychology, a training she started quite late in her life, because her first career was as an actress. At fifty, she discovered that the proportion of roles for older women in Hollywood was the reverse of the sociological reality. After a period of despair, she trained to become a psychologist at the Institute where I teach. As part of the training, she was expected to develop the basic skills: *empathy* and *listening* – at which she consistently failed. She discovered that she really could not grasp any of the emotions, feelings, or body language expressed by the classmates with which she would do the exercises. She was despairing about her future as a psychotherapist when she had a transforming experience. One day, a student in the class became so annoyed with her incapacity to listen to others, that she lashed at her: "Susan, you are such a narcissist! And you are such a drama queen! I can't team up with you anymore." At the break, Susan went into the library, to read the definition of the Narcissistic Personality Disorder (301.81):"A pervasive pattern of grandiosity (in fantasy or behavior), a need for admiration, and a lack of empathy, beginning by early adulthood and present in a variety of contexts, as indicated by five (or more) of the following nine criteria: (1) has a grandiose sense of self-importance (e.g., exaggerates achievements and talents, expects to be recognized as superior without commensurate achievements); (2) is preoccupied with fantasies of unlimited success, power, brilliance, beauty, or ideal love; (3) believes that he or she is "special" and unique and can only be understood by, or should associate with, other special or high-status people (or institutions); (4) requires excessive admiration; (5) has a sense of entitlement, i.e., unreasonable expectations of especially favorable treatment or automatic compliance with his or her expectations; (6) is interpersonally exploitative, i.e., takes advantage of others to achieve his or her own ends; (7) lacks empathy: is unwilling to recognize or identify with the feelings and needs of others ; (8) is often envious of others or believes that others are envious of him or her; (9) shows arrogant, haughty behaviors or attitudes."

She had been told that she was also a drama queen. In a state of mind Susan qualifies as an "altered state," she then read the category 301.50 of the DMS IV, the *Histrionic Personality Disorder* (which used to be called a *hysterical personality*). It has many traits in common with *Narcissistic Personality Disorder,* but has more emphasis in the need for intensity and attention (the drama queen). The eight diagnostic criteria are the following (1) is uncomfortable in situations in which he or she is not the center of attention; (2) interaction with others is often characterized by inappropriate sexually seductive or provocative behavior; (3) displays rapidly shifting and shallow expression of emotions; (4) consistently uses physical appearance to draw attention to self; (5) has a style of speech that is excessively impressionistic and lacking in detail; (6) shows self-dramatization, theatricality, and exaggerated expression of emotion; (7) is suggestible, i.e. easily influenced by others or circumstances; (8) considers relationships to be more intimate than they actually are.

Susan was in shock. She is one of the rare persons I ever met who became aware of her narcissistic/hystrionic traits, and who decided to learn a different way of relating to people. Five years after leaving the school, with her psychology degree, I met her at a conference and we talked about the day she looked at herself through the categories of the DSM IV. I asked her if we could tape an interview. I wrote a few versions of her "confession," discussed the text with her until she felt the formulation was adequate. With her permission, here is the result.

I HAD THE RAGE OF A BABY

Every partner I ever had, left me saying more or less the same thing: that I am impossible to live with. It took me a degree in psychology and years of therapy to see that I was narcissistic and hysterical–what the DSM calls histrionic. Had I been less physically attractive, and not in the acting profession, I might have discovered my problem earlier. I lived most of my life with a constant need for intravenous drips of adoration, and as an actress, I was offered that kind of adoration. Being fed a high dosage of devotion only intensified my need, like a sugar addiction that makes you crave sweets. I came to a point where I needed a drop of "You are great," every half-hour or so. Directors, camera men, sound technicians, makeup artists, all got used to compliment me regularly, otherwise I would get too nervous to perform. My personal relationships all ended because I was asking for the same kind of devotion from my lovers. The world was my stage, and my life a performance to receive applause. I didn't have eyes to see, only to check if I was seen. When I was six years old, I was already looking at myself in shop windows and claiming my mom's attention every minute of the day. At fifteen, I did a long video of myself, talking to the camera: hours of narcissistic monologue! I was present only to the image of myself, not to myself. At forty, just before losing the good looks that kept me employed as an actress, I had become so completely intoxicated with the ultra-sweet compliments I was addicted to —you look stunning/radiant/luminous/ glorious/breathtaking/ glowing/ extraordinary... that the only living creatures left to relate to were my dog and my cat. I had no friends, because I would round every situation to keep center stage, all eyes on me, my problems, my aches, my success, my needs, me at the center of everything, me the nicest flower of the bouquet, me forever planting my flag in the middle of every territory. I was blind, deaf, dumb to others, to all but me, and me again, and me all the time. I lived with the rage, the fear, the need of the child I had been, my mother's doll, her toy, her claim to fame, her compensation for a life unlived. I worked hard to become a star and I succeeded, only to discover, at 50, a big mistake in my thinking. I thought that having the adoration of a crowd would make me love myself. Mistake! What I needed to change was the way I treated others, and not the way I looked in a mirror. When I began studying to become a therapist, what really helped me was the discipline of listening to patients. I learned an openness to others that is like a daily miracle for me.

A rejection from the partner is often the necessary lesson we all need to learn: narcissism is a dangerous weed in the garden of the personality, and it needs to be uprooted on a regular basis. Had Susan decided not to hear the feedback from her classmates, her life would have turned into a typical sad story of repeated rejection and isolation. Nature is always giving us lessons about what is sustainable, and what is not. Narcissistic relationships are the ultimate example of unsustainability.

The diagnosis of narcissism was very popular in the seventies and eighties, with Christopher Lasch's denunciation of how our education system and family values breed narcissism.[95] Yet, this denunciation did not have much impact on societal policies, maybe because of Lasch's suggestion that narcissism was the result of a decline in religious practice, a theory proven wrong by further analysis. In psychology, the attention went elsewhere, and the category of Borderline Personality Disorder replaced Narcissistic Personality Disorder as the trendy diagnosis; one could be a narcissist again and nobody would notice.[96] Fads exist in psychiatry and psychotherapy, which means that a new diagnosis category offers the possibility to see something new, but also to *not see* something, once the spotlight moves away.

Post Freudians theorists such as Lacan and Kohut had a more enduring influence than Lasch, yet their ideas were expressed in a heavy jargon which was a deterrent to many. I prefer the earlier, blunt, simple affirmation by Freud and

Jung, that an adult is somebody who evolves *beyond* the primary narcissism of the child who rages at having to share mom's services. The actual widespread phenomena of adults who won't grow up, gives those approaches a new relevance, pointing at the cultural problem rather than the clinical one. Any breakup from any relationship benefits from an examination of our own narcissism which is often the "hook." As a result of the cultural tolerance for narcissism, we tend to expect from love something that is not actually possible past infancy. It creates a situation where one is never satisfied with what life has to offer, always expecting more, more, more– emotional bulimia. The cultural diet may bee too rich in sweet romance and too poor in salty wisdom.

The trophy partner: narcissism by another name
It is a great happiness, because it is a private happiness. Modesty defends every intimacy.
(Gaston Bachelard, Les Rêveries du Repos)

The healthy narcissistic component in every relationship –Freud's notion of *secondary narcissism*– makes us want our partner to look good and to reflect positively on ourselves. It is natural for parents to want to be proud of their children, and there is a legitimate narcissistic pleasure, when we buy a bigger, nicer house, to give a tour of it to our friends, feathers all fluffed up like a peacock. How many are truly beyond liking trophies, applauses and compliments? Shows of modesty are one of the preferred acts of stars, as long as the paparazzi are still pursuing them. "She/he is so simple and warm and natural," is a line journalists will use to describe a popular star *acting* modesty – until that same journalist may want to trash them. The star's modesty may be a true quality of that person, but only the intimate friends would know that. Unfortunately, it is too often an act: remove the spotlight and the need to be seen resurfaces. As we saw with Susan, narcissism may be a work-related ailment.

When the narcissistic need is the basis of an intimate relationship, the partner is mostly a "trophy," which destroys love in both partners. To say it philosophically, to be a trophy *objectifies* you; as a trophy you are a prop in the narcissist's show. In order to have a couple, or a team, persons have to be persons, not objects. If you are married to a successful and rich narcissist, and satisfied with being the trophy spouse, it may work just fine, as long as the value put on you, as trophy, is high enough. It both reveals and satisfies your narcissistic traits: to be considered an object of great value. A trophy partner usually does not get depressed at being an object, only at being a *devalued* object. It is a sad and frequent story: a man marries a beauty queen; she becomes pregnant; her body changes; she loses her sex-appeal and he loses interest in his trophy. As a consequence, she feels like garbage. Yet, her heartbreak is the occasion to become a person. Or, a woman marries a man because of his ability to make money; the money dries up and the wife stops caring for him; he feels cheated and becomes violent. His heartbreak is the occasion to find other values besides money. Or, a child prodigy wins a Chopin contest at twenty, and then decides to become a dentist; he is shunned by his narcissistic mother. His heartbreak is the occasion to discover who he is as a person.

The narcissist's display of interest in the trophy partner has very little to do with love: the partner is an item to show off to the admiring crowd. Stendhal called it *vanity love*, because that is what it is: vanity. The relationship is *not to the partner but to those others* that have the power to grant status. One indicator of a narcissistic partner is that, as soon as you, the trophy, find yourself in private with your owner, indifference replaces excitement. An intimate relationship doesn't happen on stage, which is why a narcissist lover doesn't get the point of spending energy on intimate conversations, intimate sex, intimate anything. Here is how a young man, the son of a friend, was able to smell the odor of the partner's narcissism on a cashmere coat

THE CASHMERE LABEL

Early in our relationship, my girlfriend gave me a very expensive black cashmere coat. At first, her gift made me feel that I was valued, worth the very best. Big error! Our affair had begun as a secret, because we work at the same place and I knew for sure that her supervisor, a jealous type who tried to seduce her, would make my life difficult if he knew about our affair. In the very first month of our affair, my girlfriend kept insisting that "our love" was worth the risk of losing our jobs (by which I guess she meant MY job). She was adamant: I had to "honor" our relationship enough to make it public: "I want to be able to introduce you to my friends as my partner. I am proud of you." Yet, in private, she was not so hot about me, as if, either our relationship was to be a public affair, or not at all! In public she acted as if I was a good catch, but in private, she had very little desire for intimacy. The more she insisted on coming out as partners, the more I recoiled from it, until I broke up. I gave her back the cashmere coat, to give to her next glorious catch.

A culture of consumerism is a growing ground for successful narcissists, because there are plenty of financial rewards for those who can treat persons like things. There are also plenty of individuals who are willing to remain in a miserable marriage with a narcissist, for reasons of money or power. Their marriage is a business contract: "I'll cater to your needs, as long as you pay for the services." Objectification of the Other is not something new; servants and slaves in racist societies have been or still are treated as objects, of more or less value, depending on their capacity to serve the master's needs and ambitions. Sexism should be called slavery when it allows husbands to treat their wives as property, because it is basically the same abuse: "You serve my needs and if you don't I'll retaliate, kill you or discard you with no resources."

There is nothing new, either, in the old strategy of marrying into wealth or nobility; it is not for love, but for the power attached to the name, or the money. The difference with today's culture of consumerism rests in the *clarity* of the deal; if one can say "I am marrying that person, for the glory of the name –bourgeois marrying into nobility– or for the money –aristocrat marrying into bourgeois money–, then the contract is based on a conscious choice, and an honest relationship can still exist. Whether the deal is money buying a name, or name attracting money, or money buying youth and youth attracting money, a deal is a deal, and it can be a good deal! Many a romantic courtship is a polite concealment for the commercial nature of the contract. The perversion is no so much in the deal, as in the ignorance of the real nature of the transaction. Balzac's novels describe many of the romantic baits, used by ambitious young men, in order to attract the gullible girl with a big dowry. He describes the romantic show of love, as the honey to attract the bee. The girl's parents typically negotiate back and forth, through un-romantic lawyers, to draft the financial aspect of the marriage deal. In Balzac's world, when the girl, now a wife, discovers that she was sold, her response is often to take a lover, to be a person at least with somebody. Balzac excelled at sociological realism: mix money with romance, add ambition on one side and naïveté on the other, and you have a balzacian script. When partners are not naïve, and are aware and willing to marry for other reasons than love, it is just that: a very ancient form of human transaction, not a narcissistic personality disorder, not a fraud. Many a power couple today are alliances based on values that have more to do with power (social positioning) than with romantic attraction. Respect is a frequent outcome of the clarity of their deal. Franklin D. Roosevelt had his romantic and sexual affairs on the side, yet, he knew that Eleanor was his true partner in the social and family realm; her political opinions were precious to FDR. She developed her own deep friendships on the side.[97] The same is true of many an admirable couple and it takes our culture's obsession with the romantic myth and sexual obsession, to remain blind to the value of such a conscious deal.

If your relationship with your partner was based on a power deal, it would help your recovery if you were willing to consider that the psychological damage begins not with "the deal" you both made, but rather *with the unconsciousness* about the nature of "the deal." It is the *unconsciousness*, the gullible innocence or unforgivable ignorance that is the problem, not the contractual nature of the relationship. Many women are attracted to power (usually in the form of money or fame), not love, but they don't really know the difference between those two sentiments; consequently, they expect the relationship to deliver incompatible benefits. Once married to the rich ambitious successful and busy husband, the "innocent" wife starts complaining about the husband's lack of warmth, his incapacity for intimacy, not aware that it shows her own narcissistic position of wanting to have it both ways: a wolf with competitors, a lamb with her. Her depression at being let go, has little to do with the heart and is more like the fear of unemployment. It should then be treated as such.

The same unconsciousness characterizes the tragic figure of the older man who refuses to see that his very young, very beautiful, very sexy and very ambitious trophy wife is not really attracted to him, but to his money, and that she has an hidden agenda. It is a sad thing to witness his disillusion, at discovering that the young wife has a lover on the side, or that she doesn't really care for the child she produced, in order to secure an alimony in case of divorce. Again, the problem is not so much in the deal, but, as in most interpersonal conflicts, in the incapacity to *see through* the darker aspects of the self. What becomes unbearable is not the contractual terms of the relationship (money buying youth), but the falsehood on which rests the relationship. There are plenty of examples of an older person offering financial ease, and social advantages to a younger person, in exchange for a devotion to the needs of the older partner. Nothing prevents that kind of deal from being a fair, affectionate and loving partnership. But unconsciousness and unrealistic expectations inevitably create bitter resentments. Everything that is for sale is visible, on display, and has a price. Love is invisible, private, and if it can be bought it's not love, which explains why it remains an inaccessible mystery to a narcissist. The contamination of the model of economy is clearly disastrous in the transactions of the heart.

The narcissist excels at calculating cost/benefits: "I'll give this to get that," the ultimate ability in a consumerist culture, but a cruel trap for those hungry for love. The tragedy of the narcissist is a logical one: it is a fact of our neurological makeup that a sense of self can only be built through intersubjective reciprocal interactions; but the narcissist is incapable of intersubjectivity; hence the narcissist remains deprived of a sense of self! A philosopher looking at the drama of narcissism might define the problem as such: the self is *not a thing*, it is a *no-thing, a nothingness* would say an existentialist, like love is no-thing, and joy is a no-thing. The tragedy of the narcissist is that he/she cannot relate to somebody that is not a thing.[98] Being a social success is being a valuable object in the eyes of others; that is nice, but it can never make up for the void at the core of the narcissist's personality. In terms of relating to others, the narcissist's options are reduced to a binary choice: a) the Other is an inferior being whom I can manipulate to serve my needs, or: b) the Other is a superior being, which makes me feel inferior, hence I must find the vulnerable spot to launch an attack. The narcissist cannot comprehend that there are other options, and that love can only exist between two equals, two *subjects*, not two *objects*. A narcissist is somebody who was never taught that love is an expression of our essential freedom, not something that can be put in a contract, bought, controlled, or taken by force. Most patients with a narcissistic personality disorder have lived all their life without even one model of a loving relationship; the ecosystems in which they grew up –family, school, culture– had a disturbed balance of exchange, a faulty ecology. They may have learned to relate to a partner in a business, they certainly know how to relate to an adversary, to an employee, to the objectified spouse (the spouse as part of the assets), but cannot even *imagine* how the beloved is a spiritual companion, somebody with whom to feel and create the quality of existence.

The narcissist cannot understand, either, that love comes with a moral obligation for the well-being of the other, since such a notion is the exact opposite of the principle of profitability. The narcissist understands very little of the *meaning* of the word love; his/her condition is truly the mythical curse depicted by Narcissus's tragic story: looking at himself in the reflecting pool, he fell in love with his own mirror image and never had a life. Echo, the nymph who fell in love with Echo's physical beauty, never had a life either.

A heartbreak, because it breaks the heart open, is the worst offense to whatever amount of narcissism remains in us from infancy –usually there is *a lot*! It makes a heartbreak the most precious occasion to leave behind the conditioning of our culture, that defines love as a commodity. Being rejected hurts so deeply, it rubs so hard against our natural narcissism, that it can teach us two of the most important lessons about relationships: we don't own the lover. It also can teach us to avoid being used by narcissistic manipulators, and to avoid being a narcissistic manipulator. Again, it is the *evolve or perish* message from Nature!

CHAPTER 11

REBUILDING IDENTITY

Your Beloved was the sun, the moon, the North star, the whole cosmos for your adoring eyes; together you performed a duet that occupied center stage, all the spotlights on your act, all your creativity invested in "we" and in "us." Together, you wrote the script, directed the action, funded the production, created the set and enjoyed the mutual applauds. Then, Beloved left the set, and handed you the pink slip: "Thank you very much for all the years of collaboration, I won't need your services anymore, I am taking the story in another direction, please leave the stage and recede in the dark." Here you were, like a homeless person watching the rich and the famous coming out of their limousine on Academy Awards Night, a Cinderella without a fairy godmother, a prince without a horse, a nobody, a has-been of love, an unkissed frog, just another casualty in the battle for love. This was not solitude, but isolation, rejection, sheer misery.

Real solitude is much better; it is a time to sort out what is essentially part of your identity, and what belongs to the lost identity you had with your partner. It takes tranquility and silence to rebuild a sense of self, and it takes connecting to others to test your new identity.

Mental health and relationship addiction

A teenager who spends most of his/her time collecting hundreds of "friends" on Facebook expresses the natural agony of not yet being somebody; your heartbreak has brought on a psychological vacuity similar to that of the isolated teenager. Your isolation bring with it the risk of developing a *relationship addiction,* just like so many adolescents do, because their experience was never one of healthy solitude, but rather of a painful isolation. The incapacity to remain alone necessarily leads to relationship addiction as quickly as the incapacity to relate leads to isolation. Your return to mental health requires a new balance between relating to others, and relating to yourself.

Since the ancient Greeks, not much has been written about the psychology of *mental health* because our psychiatry and psychology emerged from the medical model of *mental sickness,* whereas the Greek's notion of mental health emerged from their philosophy about the good life. We could borrow at least one of their basic principles: mental health is an equilibrium. For example, if our natural disposition is gloomy, the Greek wisdom might suggest that one should balance it by developing a comic and rosier imagination of life's dramas. The genre of comedy can be a valid counterweight to many a difficult situations. Conversely, if our natural disposition is too rosy, too romantic, and too naïve, their wisdom would recommend the study of history, and a close encounter with those who suffer tragedies. Following the Ancient Greek kind of wisdom might suggest that if you feel isolated, balance your regimen by reaching out; if you suffer from empty agitation, go for a silent retreat, or, if your social diet contains to much solitude, balance it with more relating. Traditional Chinese philosophy has a similar definition of health: a balance, or harmony between the yin and the yang. The notion of Tao, a term that literally translates as "the path", may translate as the basic energy and unity of life, which asks for balance between poles.

The values that today govern education rarely include the art of solitude, nor tolerance for silence. I find it sad, because the capacity to love implies a basic comfort with one's own quiet company. A school system (or a family) that never allows kids silence, nor solitude, creates a neurotic addiction to relationships, similar to the addiction that comes from the experience of sharing every daily routines with a partner. The "keep them busy" mentality is detrimental to the psyche; it creates a generation of kids hooked on their iPhone to communicate the most trivial information, because they can't tolerate silence. ("Hello there, I just had a hamburger. Now I am going for a walk") The more an addiction to relationships contaminates love, the more love disappoints. This neurotic aspect of symbiotic love has to be dealt with sooner or later, and mastering the art of solitude/silence is a pre-requisite to enjoy the spiritual benefits of love.

Lonely and invisible

In a heartbreak, there is a moment when you have to accept that, for the present time, you are temporarily and truly *invisible*. After all, you just lost your role in the script of your emotional life. Invisibility can be painful: peasants, serfs, slaves, servants, were always invisible for their masters. Older women today are invisible. An ex-nun told me she asked the chaplain of her community why the matriarchs in the Bible don't get as elaborate stories as the patriarchs. He didn't have an answer; she understood that in patriarchal religions women are not seen, not heard and their concerns and questions remain unanswered: they are invisible. Black characters in most of the nineteenth century American literature were invisible; the story was not about them, but about the white masters. A child in an abusive household is not seen, not heard. The low paid, untrained, disposable employee in a huge organization is invisible. As a heartbroken woman, I have inhabited the realm of the invisible. I finally had to admit my invisibility and talk to myself with the words my grandmother used to say to my grandfather, when he needed to hear an unpleasant truth: "Darling, put that in your pipe and smoke it!" I accepted my invisibility; it was extremely useful, because it cleared the stage for the next step, which is to find one's new identity.

Our identity is built through our connection to other human beings. Even the lonesome scientist, working in his lab eighty hours a week, gets his sense of self from a vocation that *in itself* connects him to the rest of humanity. One can be married to science, married to a mission, married to a cause, and these loners, although not connected to a conjugal partner, are connected to humanity. They lead beautiful generous lives, although their pursuit is solitary. Introverted artists, solo explorers, Carmelites nuns and reclusive monks are not necessarily misanthropes. Like Saint Francis of Assisi, one can walk alone in the woods, talking to the birds, and, through them little birds, reach the spiritual summit of our essential connectedness. Our relationship to others may take many forms, yet a sense of balance between solitude and connection is essential to identity formation.

A feeling of largesse starts growing anew in a mending heart; the new identity starts with a sense of belonging to this universe, of having something *to give back* to the world that gives us life. The breakup with the beloved has cut you from the world, as in the expression "He/she was the world for me" and the old identity had to dissolve in solitude before another one emerges. It seems at first that the physical absence of the beloved is the only cause of your suffering, and one is under the illusion that if he/she would only come back, all would be fine again. It is not so. There are not one, not two, but three absentees in the drama of heartbreak: the first is the Beloved; the second is the person you were *with* the beloved; and the third the person you were *for* the beloved. It is more than enough to explain the loss of a sense of identity! Individuals suffering heartbreak have nightmares of losing their nametag, passport, car keys, being lost in a strange city, walking in a cemetery and reading their name on a funeral monument, having no voice, no head, no body, coming to work and somebody else's name is on the door of their office, coming home and their mother asks them to introduce themselves ... all metaphors of an estrangement from the self. They have lost their sense of self.

If I am not myself anymore, who am I?

Neuroscience has confirmed without a doubt that love is not only a pleasurable emotion, it is one of our basic needs, like food, shelter, water. It confirms that, without loving caregivers, the human infant never develops the capacity for language and is crippled beyond repair in many more ways. One aspect of the need for love is its necessity to sustain an identity through the give-and-take of relationships. It starts as infants and never stops: "Look mom, I can walk. Look Dad, I can ride my bike. Look teacher, I got that equation right. Look professor: here is my dissertation. Look partner: here is the product of my work." The basic contract between parent and child involves all aspects of identity building: physical, psychological, social: "I am young, fragile, and I need your love to define me. I'll try to be whoever you want me to be, in exchange for your care and security. Teach me who I should be, and I'll do my best." Psychoanalysts wrote many volumes about the role of parents in the formation of the child's emerging self; and many philosophers have argued that our identity is a psycho-social construct, a compromise between what our parents want, what society wants and what we think we want, and can do best. If identity is a construct, it follows that is can be deconstructed, just like a myth is debunked (for example, the famous debunking of the myth of the divine rights of kings.) A heartbreak is a demolition derby of identity. The lover, as the mirror who used to give back a positive image, now reflects nothing, or, if it does, it is a tarnished ugly picture that communicates: "Sorry, but you are no longer loveable. Get lost!" The identity built to attract and relate to the partner is obsolete, stale, a dead cable connector. Although that deconstruction of identity is very painful, it also offers a marvelous occasion to update our connectors, to a world in constant motion. Heartbreak is such a rough deconstruction that it is not a surprise that it is felt at first like a death of the self. There is a word for that feeling: *alienation,* which means a *separation from oneself.* In the Middle Ages, the word *alienation* was synonymous with madness, the caricature of it being the lunatic patient who has so little sense of self, he thinks he is Christ, or a bird who can fly from the tenth story of the building. Sociologists later used the word *alienation* to describe any situation where the sense of self –collective or personal– is lost. For example, peasants coming to find work in the city and losing their connections to their ancestral house, culture, and mores, were said to feel alienated. Karl Marx used the word *alienation* to mean the loss of meaning in one's life, when the work does not contribute to the sense of self.

The loss of your partner is a most alienating event. You may still know you name and still perform at work, yet your core identity is shaken, the mirror broken. In order to get to that peaceful meadow, where solitude is a pleasant, calming and productive experience, one should know that the road that leads to it passes through the rough terrain of alienation.

LEA: I AM NOTHING; I AM GARBAGE!

I was married for twenty-five years. I was wife, mistress, secretary, big and little sister, confidante, confessor, guru, cook, janitor, accountant. I was his baby, his mommy, his queen, his whore and his Madonna. With the end of our marriage, all my titles are gone, all my inner characters are suddenly without substance. I am free to become whomever I wish, but I have no idea who that person should be, could do, where she should live, how, and for what purpose. I used to love reading, but I can't read; I don't know what I want to read. I used to be an active person, and now I stay in my pajamas all day, eating whatever I find in the kitchen that is still edible. Where is the person I was? Who am I supposed to be? I long for the woman I used to be, I mourn her. The truth is: I miss her more than I miss my husband. He is somewhere in the Caribbean with his new little chick. After all his lies and betrayals, I don't want him back but I am stuck in my pain; the woman I was has not yet been replaced by the woman I will be. I am not dead, but I don't seem to exist either.

Lea is in the process of letting go of an identity that *has to be left behind,* yet, in that transition, she feels like a nobody because, really, she is! Her therapy is a process of slowly discovering the person she can, and wants to be.

That process is one of *initiation,* because the change is not a simple transition from one set of activities to another. At the core of any initiation there is a letting go of the previous identity, the typical ritual requiring that the neophyte remains *in solitude*, forced to face the angst. As elements of the previous identity are stripped away, the elders, teachers or guides do not explain to the neophyte what is coming. Lost are the usual objects, places, modes of relating, in order to send the neophyte a very clear message: your past identity is gone, a new one is coming; in between, you have to remain alone with the terror of the void. The fear helps push the neophyte into the next stage of life, want it or not, because the community blocks the way back, so that there is no other way but forward. When the initiate is re-instated in the community, the new identity that emerges has more vitality than the one that was shed. A heartbreak-through follows the same process: the way back is blocked, and you have no choice but to go through periods of angst, alienation, isolation, fear of the void, tears and loss of identity. Solitude and silence are prescribed to shed the old identity and propel yourself into the next chapter of your life.

The next vignette is about a woman who called herself a "serial lover," because she had a great capacity to seduce, but not to sustain any long term relationship. When she began reflecting on herself, she did not like the person she discovered. Veronica's suicidal impulse and detestation of herself was the trigger for a needed deconstruction of her identity.

I, THE FRIGID BEAUTY QUEEN

At eighteen, I won a national beauty contest. It brought me many marriage proposals. I married the guy with the best salary. He believed that a beauty queen like myself must automatically have a warm heart and a welcoming body. He paid dearly for his illusion. For me, life was never about love, nor sex, but rather about survival. I am programmed to function in only one mode: problem solving. I have a sensual deficit. Other people around me seem to find pleasure in existing; they celebrate life, appreciate friends, fun, food, they have pleasure doing things with their loved ones. The only way I can relate to anyone is to solve their problems. I need my husband, children and parents to need me. I was sexually frigid with all my lovers, and also with the three men I married. The third husband is divorcing me for that same reason. I am technically functional, but I don't feel much, and I never, never take sexual initiative.

Veronica spent her childhood trying to support her frustrated unhappy mother, to rescue her abused grandmother, to assist her sick and overworked father, to make ends meet and to survive on a very poor farm. It hurts to see a parent suffer, so the child will carry the pain of the mother and become *mother bound*; or the child carries the

pain of the father and becomes *father bound.* Not only did
Veronica grow up to be blind to her own lack of self, she also
lived with an inner injunction that communicates: "Thou
shall not evolve past the point reached by your ancestors;
don't you dare be happier (sexier, richer, more educated)
than the people from your clan." Later, as an adult, she was
bound to offer her services instead of her love, because this
is how she had learned to relate.

*I have inherited the frigidity of a whole lineage of
heroic women, all of whom survived by denying their
material, emotional, sexual and spiritual needs. Like
my female forebears, I offered my husbands sexual
service, domestic service, secretarial service, catering
service...never risking to exist for my own sake. My
first husband left me for a woman I find vulgar and
ugly, uneducated, but, according to him, "She really
likes sex." He left me with four kids to raise, which,
of course, I did heroically. When the youngest left for
college, I met my second husband and I thought it
would be different. But soon I was back to the same
game of doing whatever he wanted. He wanted to have
another child, to insure that he and I we would be a
"real" family, thus making it quite clear that my other
four kids, because they were not biologically his, did
not qualify us as a "real family." I did not oppose that
silly egocentrism of his and I gave birth to a fifth child,*

> *which I didn't really want. The truth is: he wanted that child to tie me more securely to the hitching post of marriage. This baby-girl was like his puppy. As soon as she was old enough to argue with him he lost interest in her and he himself became my needy baby.*

Guidance from nature

If only our carrying of our loved one's pain took the burden off their shoulders, it would be sensible and generous thing to do so; when it is, the sacrifice is easy. The same is true of our devotion to fulfilling the desires and ambitions of the partner, such as the desire to start a family or have another child. Yet, because of the neurotic component in self-denial, it often does more harm than good. Many depressed patients carry over a silent injunction, formulated in a family that wordlessly communicate: "Nobody in this house should outgrow their limitations." It is the case with Veronica, whose life in the service of her husband is in fact the result of her (and his) psychological limitations. Veronica lived under the injunction that her desires (such as wanting her husband to be content with the family they already had) and her problems (constant exhaustion) were not to be considered.

> *My husband began needing more and more "servicing" because that is all I can give. Whenever I would reached burnout, which I did three times during*

that marriage, he would go for a fishing trip with his buddies, or he would have an affair with a woman less exhausted than I. I would cry myself to sleep many nights until I was back on my feet, fit for service again. He would usually promise to be faithful, to stick around on weekends, which would last until my next burnout. I divorced him, and started the same deal with the third husband. Same story and same outcome: this last husband too is divorcing me! My definition of myself as women is faulty, stupid, passé and dangerous. I am the kind of woman who, like my mother and grandmother, always chooses the piece of meat that is overcooked, leaving the best for the others, although I am the one to do all the cooking. I am stupid enough to cook gourmet meals for children who eat while talking on their cell phones —oblivious to the flavors, obvious that I am serving them. I am the kind of woman who jumps up to do the dishes while still chewing on my last bite of food, hopping on the next task. I am the kind of woman who always believes that a husband's attitude of "Wham, bam, thank you, ma'am" is perfectly natural because he is a man.

Veronica's third divorce was the first time she really let herself *feel* her alienation. She saw how thin was her identity and decided that she could change that. She had to delete the whole program working in the background, re-format her psychic hard disk and install a new identity. It was a difficult task, but a doable one. Maintaining our own sense of self in any relationship is difficult enough, but even more so when there is a regressive stance in the others around us, as there was in Veronica's milieu; she did her best to fit in their ideology, one in which education is for the rich, change is impossible and the good life is for the afterlife. Veronica never took her distance from the emotions of a period, of a culture. She was "wound identified" and needed an occasion to demolish that identification. Being left for the third time was the occasion.

> *My fundamental attitude was always to save the day! I had no revolt, even when the sex was really boring to the point of abuse. I was born to please everybody, every day, in every situation because that is what I believed is needed for a woman to survive. The slave complex! Yes, I did survive, in a sick way, by developing a maximum of control over my kids, over my husband, over the house and its content. I thought I was the perfect victim, until I looked beneath and found the huge power complex behind my victim's posturing. I did aim at dominion and my way of building a power base was by taking care of everybody and everything. Yet, I never had dominion over myself because I was satisfied with the feeling of being needed and in control. The reason I wanted control, as opposed to*

> *love, is because I was at the lowest rung of human achievement: survival. I don't have a self, how could I have a sensual self? I barely taste what I eat. I never felt love, not even for my children, and never saw the beauty in the world. I just survived. Either I become somebody, a real person, a "me," or I kill that empty shell that is me.*

A heartbreak is a form of guidance from nature: "You are hurting now, but you'll die if you pursue your old ways." The guidance is extreme, but so is nature: swim or sink, fly or crash, leave this milieu, those values, this belief, this group, this job, this Church, this city, this program, this clique, this partner... or you'll lose your vitality! Nature has no patience for either big dinosaurs or tiny molecules who can't adapt. The process of heartbreak-through is a frenzy of destruction of an identity which fails to support the evolutionary process. Traumatic learning is still learning, and each time our emotional life moves into the chaos of heartbreak, it is to stop the neurotic sabotaging that makes us sick and wastes love, because love is so crucial to survival. Letting go of outmoded, damaging forms of attachment is the real work of heartbreak. Self-identity is based on neurological circuits that are persistent but do respond to change if we are willing to retrain our brain. Even when the experiences that shaped the identity were painful, rejecting, oppressive; even when it came to feel more *natural* to live within the confined space of the fearful heart, still there is always the option to retrain the brain. On the day they are freed, long time prisoners are often afraid to leave their prison; the world seems too vast and the discovery of its beauty brings an acute misery at the thought of the wasted years, the lost life. Veronica had made herself comfortable in her domestic prison, and the intuition of all the wasted joy, the friendships avoided, the life unlived, the occasions wasted, provoked an intense fear that at first paralyzed her. Nevertheless, with the shock of a third divorce, and thanks to a period of forced solitude as well as some therapeutic help, she started rebuilding a sense of self along a different set of values. Her fear gave way to excitement and she began scrubbing clean the gluey neurotic attachment to an outdated identity.

CHAPTER 12

LOVE IN THE AGE OF IMMATURE ADULTS

Our craving inevitably creates the expectation of an Edenic condition in which the sole higher purpose is to enjoy the fruits of the earth in an increasingly infantilized state of sheer receptivity."

Robert Pogue Harrison[99]

A fairy tale typically opens with a lovely princess, safe and happy in her family's castle. In a neighboring land, there is a good-looking prince, the perfect match for such a nice princess. He is brave, although not tested yet. The adorable princess likes to make bouquets for her gentle and compassionate mother, the queen, and to befriend the animal kingdom. This kind of honeymoon with the world is what happy childhood memories are made of, or *should be* made of. As children, we should all have a chance to experience the perfect bliss of listening in sheer rapture at the tweet-tweeting birdies, strolling in the rose garden around the family dwelling, even if the flowers we pick are dandelions on the roadside, to make a bouquet for dear mom, the queen of the bungalow, while dad is the king of the Hardware Store. In the language of cinema, Act One - the first three or four minutes of the movie– depicts *the world of before*, whose existence will be challenged in the coming scenes. It shows who will have to suffer, transform, evolve and grow up. In our post-feminist culture, the genders of the archetypal love story are interchangeable: many a young man today behaves as a little princess waiting for rescue, and many a young woman is attracted by the active role of heroine. It does not change the basic script, just the genderization, as recent bluckbuster movies are found to do.

In Act Two, *evil* makes an appearance, otherwise there is no plot. Evil may take the form of a monster, or of a mean rival-king, any kind of dark Lord of the Ring will do. Inevitably the princess is shocked: "Oh No! Evil in our kingdom? I can't believe it!" Reality answers: "Yes, kiddo, there is evil in the world, time to grow up." The prince faces a similar shock, and with the courage of youth, he leaves to fight the good battle. Usually, at such a point in the story, the king and queen (mom and dad) become incapacitated, or they fall under a curse, or they are too old to fight, or, conveniently for the story to unfold, they die. Consequently, the cute princess is left to herself, and has to develop her intelligence and strength in fending off some local villains, all by herself. This part of the story is basically the demonstration of the necessity to grow up: face ordeals, take decisions and carry the consequences of those decisions. It also makes it clear that the stakes are high: life or death for the whole kingdom.

Act Three shows the victory of love, courage, competence, compassion and collaboration among all the villagers, over evil, corruption, greed and meanness. As the prince succeeds he wins the princess-cum-inheritance. They kiss, marry and the people rejoice. They become king and queen and produce the next generation for the cycle to start over again, with new villains and new heroes. Curtain!

If they fail, the story qualifies as a tragedy. Their failure means that the principle of evil has won, for all to suffer. The love between the prince and the princess symbolizes the continuation of life through the maturation of a new generation. It also symbolizes the collective values placed on peace, happiness, fertility, strength, wisdom and beauty (gardens of roses, little birds and good kids), as opposed to oppression, war, devastation, ugliness of manners and sterility. The point of telling such stories to kids is to teach them that when a prince and a princess get married, they inherit the title, the castle and the gold, but, with all that, they also inherit the responsibilities that go with their royal status. A fairy tale is the basic story about the evolution of a boy or a girl (prince and princess) into a man and a woman (king and queen). The symbol of king is the adult form of power and justice, while the symbol of queen is the adult form of love, beauty and compassion.

Sometimes the basic script is reversed, but the archetypal drama remains the same. For example, Act One may *start* with an evil force that deprives the adorable princess of the love and protection that should be hers by birthright. Scene one shows her lost in the forest, lonely, hungry, abandoned. As for the prince, scene one shows him under a curse that transformed him into a frog, a stag, a fish, a bear, or there is an usurper who has left him without land, castle and title; in other words, with nothing at all to attract a worthy princess. The narrative that starts with the principle of evil will proceed in the same way as the one that starts in paradise; both will show the trials and sufferings that are necessary in order for the prince and the princess to regain their royal dignity (their "higher self" would say a Jungian). They are helped along the way by good spirits, wise counselors, fairy godmothers (friends, teachers, therapeutic relationships), who assist in their healing. The finale is the same: regardless of their original wounding, the kids become responsible adults, and all is well that ends well in the fertile kingdom of justice and love.

Unsustainable relationships can only break

In a fairy tale, *as well in a story of heartbreak*, there is no development of the narrative, no progress, no evolution, if the protagonists remain immature and refuse to grow up. The lives of Marie Antoinette and Louis XVI, are a good example of the tragedy of a *girl*, married to a *boy*, both of them given the power of queen and king when they were still incompetent, self-centered and pleasure-seeking adolescents. Their story does not end well, as we all know!

There are other historical example of famous immaturity, for example, the often-caricatured figures of the Turkish Pasha. The word "Pasha" –from a Persian word that means "king"– originally designated somebody with a high rank in the Ottoman empire which started in the early 14th century and ended shortly after World War I, in 1923. The honorific title of Pasha was granted to governors or generals, but with the decadence of that empire, the word "Pasha" became a synonym for a self indulgent, self-serving immature potentate. It became the caricature of a king, spending his days eating and partying, enjoying absolute power over his people, and over his harem of women, all slavishly at his service, while the kingdom went to the dogs. It was, of course, a caricature, but one that exemplifies the tragedy that unfolds when an immature adult is given power to define policies, rule the land, and control the resources. Being like a Pasha, in a relationship, means that someone is entitled and spoiled; it also carries the meaning that such a character brings with it a sense of decadence in the relationship.

One has to be careful not to interpret the downfall of the Pashas as the result of their indulging in sensual pleasures. The Pashas enjoyed gastronomy, dressed in flowing silk brocade coats and feathered hats, and made love as much as they pleased, with as many women as they could afford; but so did the doges of Venice; their regal outfits and week-long partying was a sign, not of decadence, but of power, beauty and glory. The ruin or the Pashas was *not* the result of their sensual indulgence but the result of their insufferable *entitlement* , which is the main characteristic of today's immature adult. The decadent Pashas behaved as if all the richness of the empire was their due, their birthright, without having to carry any responsibility for the welfare of the people under their authority. By contrast, the doges of Venice were the builders and creators of the glory and power of their city. The Turkish Pashas were behaving like little princes and princesses, as unconscious as Marie Antoinette who, tragically, had the power of a queen and the psyche of an adolescent, one with unlimited access to dad's money and the freedom to do as she pleased.

Yet, one has to admit that we all have *Pasha moments* because we all were, or would have liked to be, daddy's little princess and mommy's golden boy, at least on some occasions, to feel aggrandized and valued. As adults, we continue to appreciate being given a break from responsibilities, protection from the powerful, and a free lunch once in a while. Regression is not, in itself, a problem, as long as it is circumscribed to its proper sphere. What woman doesn't enjoy her lover playing the rescuing hero, from time to time? And is there a man who never needed being comforted and cuddled by a woman delivering maternal care and affection? Regressive role-playing can be pleasant, and is often necessary, as long as it does not become the *unconscious default setting* in the personality, the one and only neuronal circuit working in the background, the mono-myth. When it does, the adult relationship is doomed, and a breakup is inevitable. When it does, either there is a maturation, or, if not, the cycle of falling in love and then breaking up becomes more and more destructive.

Although adolescence designates a stage in life, it is also a style of consciousness, a feeling tone, a behavioral possibility that is always present in every relationship at every moment. The energy of adolescence has both a positive and a negative value.[100] For example, the invention of contraceptive, stems from a desire to have the fun without the responsibility, just as in adolescence. The same desire provoked humans to invent not only contraceptive devices but the washing machine, the wrinkle-free garments, games, gadgets, and machines that make life *easy and fun.* Popular magazines are filled with stories of people whose money and glory allows them to remain immature without consequences; it helps us dream: "If only I had that kind of money, I sure would indulge in…" The advertising industry is based on the fact that having money to spend is universally attractive, because it offers the seductive option of remaining like a spoiled and irresponsible child. Boys with gray hair, menopausal princesses, Marie-Antoinettes on their dad's –or their husband's–credit card, all are willing to gulp the message from their TV: "Indulge, you are worth it."

There is a very good side to our dreams of passivity, but only if we can differentiate them from the self-indulgence of the immature adult. The "good" passivity is a *capacity to receive*; without it, we could not, past infancy, trust anybody to take care of any of our needs. What a lonely destiny that would be! Those whose trusting capacity was harmed, don't get much pleasure from being served breakfast in bed, from being supported, hugged, fed, helped, taught. It is one of the pleasure of love to feel that our needs, at least occasionally, are met by the partner, because love can only be *given* or *received*, like grace; it cannot be bought. Our delight in passivity comes with our biological makeup, which allows us to experience the sensuality of human exchanges. A *capacity to receive* is a magnificent gift from life. Taoism calls it the *yin principle*. Individuals whose *yin* is underdeveloped, suffer from a reduced sensual experience. Their moments of passivity have a *mistrustful* quality, which psychology calls a passive/aggressive temperament: "I depend upon you for my pleasure, and I *resent* you for it."

Nevertheless, despite the fact that it is delightful and essential to enjoy being at the receiving end, every normal human being *also* wants to develop the opposite principle, the active principle which *controls* these sources of pleasure. Taoism calls it the *yang principle*. Neuroscience defines this active principle as the basic neocortical push toward ever more cognitive development. Freud symbolized the same active principle by his theory of penis envy, Lacan by the phallus, Jung by the animus, and Joseph Campbell by the hero's journey. Philosophers consider it one of the core value of all humans worth their salt, and discuss the active principle under the rubric of the human quest for freedom. The active, yang, heroic principle is what is needed to take active steps in one's destiny, instead of remaining a passive victim. Again, let's not forget that symbolization by biological gender (like Freud's penis envy, Jung's animus, or Campbell's hero) has lost much of its metaphorical appeal in post-feminist cultures, because it is now quite acceptable, without risking shunning, to be a yin man and a yang woman. Postmodern and post-feminist cultures are comfortable with the idea that the passive/ active polarity is present in every human, male or female. Instead of *penis envy*, I call it *action envy* ; it is an urge to fight one's battles, to influence our destiny by choosing the myths to live by. That urge is, in girls no less than in boys, the same fundamental desire that pushes the child to leave the nest. It does not invalidate the archetypal nature of those polarities. As Susan Rowland[101] has shown, one can still be interested in Jung's polarization of the anima and animus, and remain a feminist.

Falling in love begins with the delight of passivity, the honeymoon being a culmination of the passive pleasure of being loved, cherished, and pampered by the partner– "You're my baby and I love you." Sweet sweet moments! In a heartbreak, the individual is radically and suddenly deprived of all passive pleasure, of protection and of support. As we have seen throughout this book, such a trauma reactivates in the brain the fear of the powerlessness that defines infantile passivity. A baby can only *receive*, and any disruption in the service is felt as a death threat. In a heartbreak, one feels again that dark impotent aspect of passivity; it is an involuntary regression, and this time the regression is not a pleasurable one, with none of the fun of being at the receiving end, when what was delivered were flowers and kisses. There is a way to stop being the passive victim of the partner's: call back the adolescent in you, its energy and will to separate. Adolescence represents the archetypal effort to break free of the parents' control and expectations. It is a difficult task, because, at the same time as the active principle is activated for the first time in one's life, the adolescent would also like to keep the benefits of a dependent: "I refuse your authority, but could I have free room and board in the family home"? The experience of adolescence is a long stretch of clashes of expectations between parents and adolescents. The adolescent wants to get a life, but does not want to work and pay for it. Those push and pull between dependence and autonomy re-appear with more or less intensity in all adult relationships, and they reappear with acuteness in a heartbreak. The more there is immaturity in the relationship, the more intense was the competition for who gets to remain the spoiled child and who bears the responsibilities. If you were the provider/nurturer you now feel cheated and burned out, but this feeling will end as soon as you let go of the immense power attached to the role of Official Nurturer and adopt your self as your main responsibility. If your position before the breakup was the cherished princess, you felt controlled, house-bound, imprisoned in a harem. In both cases, a breakup forces evolution. Give a chance to this adolescent figure that still lives in your psyche; feel the torment you felt in adolescence: wanting to break free, move out, get a new identity, go through initiation to discover a new dimension of love. And the good news is that, as an adult, you have more resources than you had at the time of adolescence to break free. Once your realize this fact, it becomes easier to take responsibility for your needs.

To love is to support and cherish each other, but without entrapping each other. An immature adult has not yet learned that kind of relating. Marie Antoinette and the Pashas were historical figures, who were good illustrations of the damage done by immature adults. Here is another portrait of the person *you don't want to be*, through a critique of psychology.

A marvelous misfortune

Alice Miller's book, *The Drama of the Gifted Child* [102] published in the seventies, was probably the epitome of a psychology that looked at the problem of the clashes of expectations between parents and children, but exclusively from the point of view of the child. By siding unilaterally with the point of view of the child, she was the typical product of a psychology that is itself too often caught in a unilateral world view: that of the child. To give her credit, Alice Miller documented the real problem of a child who has to carry extremely heavy parental projections: "I want you, my son, to become an engineer because I could not." Her theory points at a basic and important reality, formulated earlier by Jung. He pointed out how one of the greatest burdens a child must bear, is the unlived (unconscious) life of the parents. Alice Miller popularized the notion by showing how crippling it can be for the child to be expected to fulfill the parent's fantasies. She further elaborated on what she called the child's *dark secret*, a complaint that sounds somehow like this: "I am not really myself, I am my parent's fantasy; their love is fake, I was never loved for my *real self*, but for my capacity to manifest their ideal. Their projections are my prison, and if I come out of that prison, I will lose their love, however fake it is, and that is why, poor little me, I still don't know who I am... etc...." What this kind of theorizing fails to see, is that the inner crippled child is an *archetype*, not a sickness of the psyche. It means that the frightening task of having to find one's own identity is unavoidable. For sure, there can be abuse when the parent's projections are overbearing, but there is no *dark secret*, just the normal painful process of growing up. Alice Miller, like most of the theories that aimed at saving the "inner child" started with the best of intentions. In Miller's case it was a legitimate desire to counteract the Germanic harsh abusive childrearing practices, that were the norm in her youth, and of which she was a victim. Today, it might be the Tiger Mom[103], who attracts a similar criticism. Miller's outrage at the way children were educated was a useful denunciation. Unfortunately, it created a supplementary handicap; many adult patients, reading Miller, took it as a permission to remain childish: "How dare *anyone* have *expectations* about me? I have been robbed of my *true self*, and I have a right to feel cheated, angry, and a victim." Although it was not a deliberate intention, Alice Miller's psychology of a child's *true self* fueled the business of victimology for a whole generation of educators and psychotherapists. What, one might ask, is the *true self* of a child? No child, ever, had the capacity to determine, apart from the family and the culture, an independent sense of self. Certainly, a boy should be able to express "I don't want a baseball bat, I want a violin" and a parent worthy of that title, should be respectful of those early expressions of a talents and preferences. Yet, it does not mean a child is in position to know his/her *true self* without some hardship. Finding one's identity and developing one's unique talent, is a though task, one that is indeed more difficult if the parents are self-centered, themselves busy with finding their *true self*, but a task that is part of the process of maturation.

The model of the wounded inner child is useful only if it comes with a caveat, one that the Ancient Greeks would have found so obvious as to not even make a psychology out of it: *we are all wounded and we are all victimized by life's hardships, one way or another.* We are *all* born vulnerable, incompetent and fragile, with no real sense of self; the human beings responsible for our care can never be perfect; they are often incompetent, limited and busy with other tasks and other priorities. If your caretakers were abusive, stupid, evil, obtuse, or holding beliefs that poisoned your early childhood, your task is daunting, but still possible. That the world is imperfect and contradictory, is the premise with which we start developing a sense of self and a capacity for freedom. What breeds despair is not necessarily the severity of the trauma, nor the difficulty of the task of growing up, but what the person fails to do *for herself*, as well as the capacity of the milieu to offer alternatives for abused children. The French psychiatrist, Boris Cyrulnik[104], has spent his career demonstrating how resilience is helped when a culture supports the human need to evolve beyond one's wounding and offers help to move away from victimization. He calls some hardships– including his own, as a war orphan– a *marvelous misfortune*. Indeed, misfortune can be marvelous when it forces the child to develop new strengths. His approach is at the opposite spectrum of Alice Miller's psychology; Cyrulnik focuses on developing resilience, while Miller insist on the victimization.

Think of your heartbreak as one such *marvelous misfortune*. The feeling of victimization is undeniable: it temporarily deprived you of the sense of self you fought so hard to acquire. It wiped out your whole emotional map: you were left with no location and no direction! It deprived you of all passive delights and it made you feel as powerless as in childhood, and as conflicted as in adolescence. Nevertheless, call it a *marvelous misfortune* and see how you can create resilience with it. Carol Pearson[105], in her description of the orphan archetype, summarizes the orphan's basic life complaint in a simple formula: "See how I suffered" but also: "See how I survived." Like Cyrulnick, she insist that the gift of the orphan archetype can be resilience.

One of the most dangerous pitfalls in all situations of heartbreak and mourning is to fall into self-victimization, projecting on the absent spouse, the figure of the abandoning parent which makes you the poor victimized orphan. Those who take the road of self-pity deprive themselves of their adult freedom.

CHAPTER 13

A LIBERATION OF THE HEART

[...] People brought their sorrows and perplexities, and besought her counsel, as one who had herself gone through a mighty trouble. Women, more especially, - in the continually recurring trials of wounded, wasted, wronged, misplaced, or erring and sinful passion, - or with the dread burden of a heart unwieldy, because unvalued and unsought, - came to Hester's cottage, demanding why they were so wretched, and what was the remedy! Hester comforted and counseled them, as best she might. She assured them, too, of her firm belief that, at some brighter period, when the world should have been ripe for it, in Heaven's own time, a new truth would be revealed, in order to establish the whole relation between man and woman on a surer ground of mutual happiness.

Nathaniel Hawthorne [106]

Up to this chapter, we have seen how the principles of recovery from heartbreak recapitulates many of the most fascinating discoveries of neuroscience, among which are the demonstration of how:

a) our brain reacts to the quality of our milieu,
b) is influenced by the level of our intellectual activity,
c) responds to the atmosphere of interpersonal exchanges,
d) is hungry for new learning,
e) can evolve quickly, when facing adversity, leaping forward in a surprising evolutionary jump,
f) or can regress and degenerate as quickly, when deprived of stimulation and challenges.

Neuroscientists are telling us, in a nutshell, that, depending on the milieu, the brain either evolves or regresses, what some call the "use it or lose it" theory.[107] Those who live in a rigid cultural milieu, one that is closed to new ideas, with few challenges and little opportunity for new friends or new world views, curb the development of their brain because the brain will adjust to a low stimulation by a minimal development of neuronal connections. If, on the other hand, the life-situation changes drastically and creates new challenges – a *marvelous misfortune* would say Cyrulnick– there is an activation of the learning centers of the brain. Contrary to the Darwinian theory of slow evolution, it is now accepted that the brain's capacity to adapt is much quicker than was formerly imagined, but *only if* the environment offers challenges and options. Evolution has been shown to be stepwise, not so linear, and the brain to be capable of quantum leaps[108]. The enduring Nature/Nurture controversy seems to have come to rest by the admission of the equality of both principles, at least when mammals are concerned. As Jaak Panksepp writes: "Thus, while basic emotional circuits are among the tools provided by *nature*, their ability to permanently change the life course and personalities of organisms depends on the *nurturance,* or lack of nurturance, that the world provides."[109]

We have seen also how neuroscience has definitively established the fact that we think, feel, imagine with our *whole body*, and not just with the brain. Descartes' mind-body dichotomy is definitely not as useful as it was when he formulated it, in order to justify the separation of science from religion. Not only do we think and feel with our whole bodies, we think and feel either *in unison*, or *in conflict* with the world surrounding us. Both the unison and the conflict are formative. No one will ever again be able to argue that the physiological events happening in the brain are independent from what is happening in our relationships, at the work place, in our culture. The brain-versus-culture dichotomy is as passé as the Cartesian dichotomy of mind-body. Our brain is definitively shaped as much by the evolution of relationships and the culture we live in, as it is by climate or diet. The relationship between culture and brain is a feedback loop: culture is shaped by the brain, the brain is shaped by culture. That is why your milieu and the *ideas* you entertain about love and relationships influence your recovery from heartbreak. The many heartbroken individuals who slowly deteriorate, and live the rest of their life with a scarred and scared heart, are those who remain isolated in a culturally poor and ideologically rigid community, offering only one way to think about love– the traditional one, belonging to the past. All the individuals I have seen break free of the inner prison of heartbreak, had taken up the challenge, tried something difficult, learned new patterns of relating to the world, to friends, to lovers, and found a way to intensify the neocortical learning centers. Healing from a heartbreak is as big a jump as the passage from adolescence to maturity, and with many similarities. The natural process of maturation is not something that happens once and for all, it is always happening. A heartbreak precipitates the need for another step in this process of maturation, and one should be grateful when it happens.

William, a year after getting his Ph.D. in psychology, sat with me to express, in the words of psychology, the gift that was his heartbreak.

WILLIAM, A YEAR AFTER HIS SUMMER IN EUROPE

With hindsight, I find my heartbreak with Laura was the one period of my life when my instinct was the most disconnected from my mind. Laura could not, nor could I, understand how we were both reacting from our complexes. Her lack of empathy toward me on the morning when I went to her apartment to deliver her mail, only to be treated like an intruder, was the most humiliating moment of my life. This humiliation was a valuable blow to my ego, because it brought down all my defensive walls. Had I known more about myself–

or about psychology— I would have known, right then, that our separation was inevitable, given both our parental projections on each other. I have learned that much: an intense parental projection on the partner kills a lover's connection quicker than hatred! I did not see how I activated Laura's complexes, and she could not see I felt like an abandoned child. Breaking each other's heart was a necessity, a most valuable lesson about matters of the heart. I prefer the heart I have now, more than the heart I had then. Paradoxically, I am grateful for the heartbreak.

A successful heartbreak-through

The kind of psychology that is now developing in association with neuroscience reveals the vast collective libidinal economy that holds together the whole system of human relations. It connects anew the brain and the poetical notion of the heart. Just like the yogini pays great attention to the body's posture while meditating, if you give yourself the right conditions, your brain will work day and night to get you unstuck from the stagnation of heartbreak. A crocodile cannot learn and a pup cannot bear to be left alone. But your human cortex is telling you: "The partner's return is a mountain you have to stop trying to conquer with a flag of your colors. Point toward the other summit: freedom. Move away from the lyrical, sticky, gooey misery of your passive defeat; use the violence of your heartbreak to break the magnetic spell that keeps you in bondage."

There is an element of uncertainty in all interpersonal relationships, as there is in our relationship to Nature; just as we cannot predict the long term climatic conditions, we cannot predict the evolution of any given relationship. At times, it is wise to accept that whatever is happening in a relationship will just keep happening, like a storm which takes it course; the partner breaking your heart is like Nature doing its thing. The Beloved could not help hurting you, just like a snow storm can't help causing a traffic jam on the roads. The sting of betrayal soon feels like the sting of a particularly cold winter.

A *successful* heartbreak enhances our sense of the interconnectedness of all human beings, like a fast restores appetite. With time, the painful aloneness is replaced by the art of keeping good company with oneself, and offers as well a wider spectrum of connecting possibilities with the rest of the world. I find that the biography of Eleanor Roosevelt shows an example of a truly successful heartbreak. Early in life, she suffered the worst of all heartbreaks, which is the loss, absence, or rejection by our first great love, Mommy dearest and daddy dearest. Young Eleanor was not pretty, did not look good in frilly dresses and lacked the feminine social charm her mother so naturally exuded. Her mother's death, when Eleanor was only eight years old, and soon after, the disappointment of discovering that the father she so admired was an alcoholic who died in an institution, were traumatic events that could break anybody's spirit.[110] Yet her heartbreak turned into the kind of *heartbreak-through* that is a possible positive outcome for all heartbreaks. At first, she was greatly helped by the headmistress who contributed to her education, in a college for girls in England; this woman helped her move away from the family tragedies and develop a sense of competence in service to society. From there, she developed her unique identity, using every negative situation to become a stronger person. She became one of the most cherished figures in the history of American politics.[111]

An *evolutionary jump*, after a trauma, is possible only if one understands that the recovery process is not a *getting back to normal*, not a return to the person one was with the partner, because the definition of what feels good and "normal" has to change. Like a mutation, or like developing immunity to a psychological virus, a new identity must emerge. For Eleanor, the resolution of her heartbreak meant accepting that she would never be the charming, elegant woman that the spirit of the time wanted her to be. She had to find who else she could become in order to feel good about herself. To move out of being the shy and isolated girl, she had to mourn the myth of parental love, which says that mom and dad's love is a given. Not so for Eleanor! She also had to deconstruct the sentimental lies and cultural clichés of her time about womanhood. This first heartbreak helped her deconstruct clichés about marriage, and made her capable of a great political partnership with her husband.

Love, of course, is a basic building block of the brain, yet Neuroscience confirms the impact of *everything* in our milieu: the quality of *all* our relationships (like that teacher who helped the adolescent Eleanor). The quantity and quality of our neuronal connections depends on everything that constitutes our psycho-cultural milieu. Yet, neuroscience does *not* say that changing the brain is easy, we often need to be pushed in the direction of change by some major threat, such as a heartbreak.

Many new theories that pervades the neuroscientific[112] and infant research literature[113] are consistent with findings in cognitive neuroscience that demonstrate how the mind emerges from neuronal interactions with other humans. In the jargon of systems theory, were are *nested systems,* which mutually influence each other. In simple terms: your therapist, your teacher, your friends, can have as big an impact on your life as the original caregiver, and as the partners that have shaped your perspective on life. This idea confirms many of the Jungians assumptions about psychological life, especially Jung's notions of the collective unconscious, which fits with contemporary notions of nested and interacting systems.[114] The connection between brain and culture is not one of strict causality, but rather the result of a mutual interaction within nested systems out of which *emerges* what we call the culture, or the environment, the personality. Hence a model of *emergence* as opposed to the old causal model: we all *emerge* from a culture in which we contribute our talent (or lack of it). Neurogenesis (what lives in our brain) is truly the epitome of an interactive process, a co-creation.

Our wonderful capacity for change, based on the malleability of the brain, can be used for the worse, as in brainwashing techniques. The capacity for change and learning may also remain only a capacity, as in the case of children raised in isolation, whose vocabulary never reaches more than a dozen words. By the same process, an individual can remain stuck for years in the pain of heartbreak; neurogenesis can fail to happen because the past neuronal organization (the connection to the departed partner) has too strong a claim on the brain.

CONCLUSION

The work of the psychotherapist is always shadowed by feelings of inferiority which fasten on the fact that he or she is "not medical." To come to its own, psychotherapy has to stand apart from its medical oppressor who speaks with the voice of materialism, scientism, and linear causality.

James Hillman

For somebody such as myself, who has spent all my adult life as a depth psychologist, it is nice to find that neuroscience confirms a great many of the assumptions of my discipline. Yet, it does not mean that these two fields have the same approach: their methods are completely different and should not be confused. The symbolic and the medical are not contradictory visions, they are the confirmation, from neuroscience itself, that our human bodies are *not only* biochemical organisms situated in space and time; we are permeable to our cultural and interpersonal environment. Again, in non-ambiguous terms, neuroscience demonstrates how the conversations we have, the books we read, the films, the songs, the ideas, the friends, the architecture of our houses, the beauty or ugliness of our cities, the climate, the symbols, the stories, the values, the ideologies, religions and myths we live by... all contribute—or fail to contribute—to building new synaptic connections that make us who we are, who we become, how we evolve and thrive, or regress and get sick[115].

Neuroscientists have been able to *explain* how the brain's plasticity (its capacity for neuronal reconfiguration) depends on our capacity to *imagine* and then to *try* new ways of being. Science has demonstrated the necessity of a rich inner life for the health of our neurons; yet, delivering that rich inner life is not a prerogative of science. In other words, neuroscience, per se, cannot open our imagination, deepen our psyche, produce symbols; that capacity belongs to relationships, to art, to depth psychology and to the humanities. Just like the explanations I once gave to the retired professor to teach him to swim, science can *explain* the processes happening in our brains, but only the emotional direct experience of immersion will have an impact on the brain. All our lives, even at an advanced age, we can, if we are willing to make the effort, learn new tricks and find inspiration that moves us to change. True enough: you can't teach new tricks to an old dog! But humans are not dogs, and old healthy humans, just like somebody suffering heartbreak, can learn new modes of being.

There is an ongoing debate between scientists: on one side are the neuroscientists who call themselves the "connectionists" and who see the brain as a "ready-to-respond-to-environment" kind of machine; on the other side are the neuroscientists who describe the brain as made up of "ready-to-access" modules that the environment merely stimulates. However, what is of interest for the healing of heartbreak is not where they disagree, but where they all agree, which is to confirm that we are *not* prisoners of our genes; and that we are *not* slaves to the processes happening in our brains. In the words of John Ratey: "The majority of neuroscientists see a hybrid, where the broad outlines of the brain's development are under genetic control, while the fine-tuning is up to the *interaction of brain and environment*. [...] Our own *free will* may be the strongest force directing the development of our brains, and therefore of our lives." [116] The notion of *free will* is one of those big philosophical questions that is relevant to the healing process because it means that *you have to want to heal*; wanting to heal has to be an expression of your free will. Otherwise, you'll remain in the emotional limbo of heartbreak, waiting for a kind of reparation that is unlikely to happen, even if your partner was to return.

A generation ago, scientists and humanists agreed with the evolutionary biologist Edgar Wilson, who wrote in 1988 : "There has never been a better time for collaboration between scientists and philosophers, especially where they meet in the borderlands between biology, the social sciences, and the humanities. [...] We have the common goal of turning as much philosophy as possible into science" [117](pp. 11-12). I find that such a worthy goal can be reversed, and it still makes sense: "Our common goal is to turn as much science as possible into philosophy." It seems to me that both the medical and the symbolic participate in the liberation of the heart. One has to develop a scientific understanding of the processes happening in the brain, *and* one has to acquire a new philosophy of love. As for that borderline between depth psychology and neuroscience it is that place in which healing from heartbreak asks for a revision of everything one *does, thinks, feels, expects, believes,* about love and about the brain.

The advance in the neuroscientific mapping of the brain has allowed the general public to understand the degree to which love is a biological foundation for the development of emotional as well as cognitive abilities; it has explained how, when love is abruptly denied, we are emotionally and cognitively impaired; it demonstrated how, at the beginning of our lives, the search for love is an *instinct*, part of the survival instinct, as much as the search for food. Neuroscience has also explained how even an instinct can fail to develop, as is the case with unloved little monkeys, kittens, puppies, or rats. Neuroscientists have demonstrated, first in their laboratory, then in the natural environment, how mammals develop an "attachment neurosis" that renders them incompetent parents, problematic partners, or isolated individuals with suicidal behaviors.[118] Studies of adult couples show, without a doubt, how our early relationship to the caregivers will emerge again as problems in the relationship to the partner.

Many neuroscientists, like Hofer and his colleagues, do their research with laboratory animals, which means that their research can inform us only about the mammalian aspect of heartbreak. Another neuroscientist, Jaak Panksepp, needed to remind the scientific community that what is true of laboratory rats may be much more complicated for humans[119]: neuroscientists are faced with the fact that, for humans, the search for love is more complicated than for other mammals. The pain of heartbreak would have had a medical solution by now, if love were *only* an instinct. As a matter of fact, there are already chemical solutions for the part of our heartbreak that is limited to the mammalian brain.[120] Unfortunately, although anxiolytic and antidepressant drugs can help with many of the physiological underpinnings of the trauma, there can't be a complete medical solution to heartbreak. Although dogs, dolphins, and elephants do experience heartbreak, the resolution of *human* heartbreak involves all aspects of our humanity, including the moral and spiritual dimensions of loving another free human being. As a psychologist, working with humans rather than with animals, my task, very different from that of a neuroscientist, is to take the problem where science leaves it, and foster recovery where medicine is powerless.

Neuroscience is presently one of the most exciting areas in science, one that promises to deliver the cure for such ailments as Alzheimer's disease, autism, and schizophrenia, all of which appear related to problematic brain chemistry or configuration. Nevertheless, as a psychologist, one has to be cautious, because these same developments in neuroscience are also responsible for the overmedication of millions of children and adults, who become addicted from infancy to drugs for all kinds of ailments, that may stem from psycho-cultural problems. A generation ago, psychology was guilty of suggesting that schizophrenia and autism were the result of faulty mothering. This was a tragic misconception for the many parents who spent their lives trying to adjust their behavior to cure their child, and it created a lot of unnecessary guilt. Schizophrenia and autism, as we now know, are the result of a brain dysfunction, not the result of a psychological trauma. Today, we are faced with the reverse danger: the medicalization of many a psychocultural dis-ease. It never was and never will be easy, to differentiate a problem which is strictly neurobiological from one which expresses a cultural dysfunction, because, as neuroscience itself is demonstrating, the brain emerges from culture and culture emerges from the functions of the brain. Big Pharma is always ready to offer medication for whatever appears to be sickness. Heartbreak is the perfect example of the kind of sickness that calls for explanations from neuroscience, *but also* calls for a revision of our cultural expectations about love and relationships. Both!

Depth psychologists have something in common with the Dalai Lama: a fascination with the concordance between the findings of neuroscience and the insights acquired by wise men and women of diverse spiritual disciplines. While neuroscientists sometimes appear arrogant, as if they were the ones who discovered the notion of the unconscious, or that meditation calms the mind, or that metaphors influence perceptions, their approach offers the scientific *explanation* that was lacking. Long before neuroscience, it was common knowledge that a child born without hands coulf be taught to use his toes to accomplish tasks beyond what a person with hands cold do. Yet, we did not know exactly *how* to explain this plasticity of the brain. Similarly, we have always known that a blind person will compensate by developing acute hearing; and we have always known that a child deprived of love won't develop. No surprise there! What neuroscience has contributed is a detailed *understanding* of *how* something as ethereal and invisible as meditation, love, compassion, ideas, and education can actually modify the physical structure of our brains. Neuroscientists are terribly impressed with their discovery: Oh wow! Intangible emotions *do* modify the synaptic connections! Depth psychologists, and the Dalai Lama as well, are impressed with the biological proof, of the non-dualistic aspect of our nature. We feel confirmed that although the mind is ethereal and the brain is physical, both have real impact on our lives.

Neuroscientific research takes place in labs, most of the time with animals, but more and more often with humans, using Functional Magnetic Resonance Imagery (fMRI), or by slicing dead brains into thin layers to fit under the microscope, or by analyzing the behavior of brain-injured individuals, or by producing new evidence through experimental testing. The scientist works in the lab, the monk meditates, the therapist listens to stories; science is science, meditation is meditation, psychotherapy is psychotherapy. Yet, these differing approaches share a common fascination with the human potential for healing or for self-destruction.[121]

The fact that the brain can be trained, is sometimes confused with a kind of New Age trend that borrows from quantum physics and neuroscience, only to create a mythology of unlimited ego power. It is not the fact that these claims are presented with reference to science, but rather that the scientific discoveries—such as the law of attraction, the plasticity of the brain, or the dual nature of waves and particles—are interpreted to *mean* something that the research is not meant to mean. That *something* is usually an ego-boosting message that caters to the culture of narcissism: "Here is the cosmos and here is your marvelous brain. Tap into its power to attract health, wealth, love, success and longevity"! Some, but not all, of these New Age gurus use words such as evolution, higher consciousness, higher self, visualization, manifestation, positive thinking and psychic energy, while omitting the most crucial part for anybody truly interested in gaining consciousness: the absolute necessity of examining the possibility of failure, the dark emotions, the regressive pulls, and the discipline needed to obtain results—in other words, at everything that asks for a real learning process with commitment and effort. What some of these pseudo-gurus are really selling, with great commercial fanfare, is the blissful ignorance of hurt and evil, and an infantile dream of easy abundance and godlike power. Their relentlessly optimistic suggestions that anybody can access the healing superpower of the brain, come with a view of the cosmos imagined as our own personal playground. It confuses the self (as Jung understood it) with the ego, and has very little to do with a true process of transformation, and much to do with the consumerist aspect of the culture.

I must add a caveat: first, all those who are now considered New Agers are not necessarily guilty of such inflation, and, second, the definition of New Age is often made by the media and is frequently unreliable. An author can be labeled as *New Age* because he/she is interested in the spiritual dimension of the psyche, as Jung was. Jung himself is still considered as a New Age author by some of his critics, which reveals a terrible confusion between genres.[122] My critique of New Age stems from a sense that a positive outlook should never exclude an examination of the darker aspects of our nature. It is also a critique of much of the self-help literature that has a much impact as a New Year list of good resolution: nil! The brain does not oblige to transform only to please the ego. It will transform only if you are broken enough that either you evolve, or you regress and die. Self-help literature is not, in itself, a bad thing, it can be educational, but the "food for thought" it offers may be too low on protein, or, in the worst cases, like a fast-food industry, not so good for your psychological health. The best judge in your own critical sense.

Jungian psychology, or for that matter, Buddhism, are forms of wisdom that suggest an attitude opposite to New Age self-aggrandizement—an attitude of humility. It teaches that a heartbreak makes you a vulnerable, neurotic, pitiful, love-obsessed, defensive, heartbroken human. It suggest that a spiritual journey starts with an honest examination of one's shadow and regressive infantile whishes. The Jungian concept of *individuation*, with its extensive examination of one's hidden darkness, is totally opposed to the kind of New Age grandiosity, a snake oil for the psyche, sold to gullible consumers. Somewhere between the two extremes of self-inflation and self-hating, there is a place where life is possible, and that is the kind of wisdom that you'll find once your heartbreak becomes a breakthrough and is remembered as the *marvelous misfortune* it can be.

* * *

As I proofread the last version of this book, I was seated in an airplane beside a cute six-year-old boy, traveling alone, his name written on an ID card hanging around his neck. He asked me if the plane, since it goes so fast, would soon reach the horizon. I would have liked to explain that the horizon is something like *pure love*: we keep flying in its direction, but as a final destination, it can never be reached. Yet without the horizon of love, human life would have no meaning and no sense of direction. Instead, I did my best to give the boy as much of a scientific explanation as a six-year-old can grasp: the curvature of the earth, the optical illusion... but clearly, it was the *experience* of this phenomenon which fascinated him, not so much the scientific *explanation*. Same for love: neuroscience can *explain* love, but what really fascinates us is the *experience*, one which needs to be preserved at all costs, above and beyond the pain of heartbreak. That pain turned your world into a horrible place, so you would be pushed out of the limited cage you believed was your love nest. Let those redeeming tears flow, and the fragile butterfly of the soul will come flying; your pain can help you become more fully human. As you'll leave the confines of your romantic illusions, you'll see the immensity of the possibilities of a life well lived, you will feel the immensity of the human heart.

We have in our hearts whole cities, peopled with all kinds of ghosts. Most of us are familiar with the ghosts of our deceased parents, lovers, friends, who still visit us in our dreams, reviving our love for them, or sometimes provoking unexpected fresh anger, even when they have been dead a long time. We are less familiar with other kinds of ghosts: for example, the ghost of the person one might have become, if love had been offered in a different manner; or the ghost of a lover whom, we feel with certitude, could have been our soulmate, but life's circumstances prevented it; or the ghost of a friend to whom we opened our heart only to be betrayed; or the ghost of a partner we stopped loving; or, most painful of all, the ghost of a child once happy, joyous and loving, who turned into a self-centered adult incapable of loving, nor working. Even in the most enduring love story, we are not spared the experience of a partner who, for a short or long period, becomes cold, withdrawn, indifferent, busy elsewhere, the ghost of the person we fell in love with. We visit with all these ghosts in dreams, and we confront them when forced by the pain of heartbreak.

Joy and Sorrow are the two priestesses that meet us at the gate of the rich inner city called "*me.*" The priestess by the name of Joy greets us with these words: "I am Joy. I defend the eternal principle of Love, no matter what, because if Love were to die, I too would die, and humans would not survive the catastrophe." Joy stands side by side with her unavoidable twin sister, the priestess by the name of Sorrow, who has this to say: "I too defend Love, which cannot exist without me. I am Sorrow, who creates the need for Love." As I entered their territory, they said in unison: "Take it all, or leave it all."

ADDENDUM

UPDATING THE TRIUNE
THEORY OF THE BRAIN

MacLean's triune theory of the brain entered the general public in the 1970s and '80s by the astronomer Carl Sagan and the novelist Arthur Koestler and it showed up recently in a popular book, *A General Theory of Love,* by Lewis, Amini, Lannon (2000) explaining the anatomical structure that we call love.

MacLean believed in a kind of "directional evolution" as if human beings were forever evolving toward a better brain. The problem with this optimistic view is that it is inconsistent with recent understanding of the evolutionary process that demonstrates how, under certain circumstances, our brains could also adapt in a way that is a lessening of our potential. His critics remind us that the theory of evolution does not imply that our adaptations are necessarily a progress, and that at any time we could become stupider and stupider, fall into a Dark Age of the brain, lose some of our intelligence. As Butler and Hodos, (2005, p. 116) remind us, "this unidimensional progression, seemingly under the direction of some imperative, is reminiscent of the now discredited, 'predetermined path' theory of apparent steady lines of 'progressive' evolution or a trend in one definite direction, referred to as orthogenesis . It can be an adaptation, a regressive one, and it is more frequent than we would like to believe. "

The same authors formulate another frequent critic of MacLean's triune theory has to do with the way he conceived of the three brains as three different stages of evolution: " [...] the critical weakness of MacLean's model is his description of brain evolution as a ladder like process of progressive change and his invocation of three 'directional evolution, views that are inconsistent with modern understandings of the evolutionary process" (Butler & Hodos, 1996).

This critique is well taken, and can be interpreted to mean: beware, you can adapt to your heartbreak by becoming a fearful, mean, egocentric, depressed individual incapable of ever loving again. Psychotherapists see that sad phenomenon regularly: individuals who react to loss by becoming passive, depressed and rigid. They have adapted to a loveless life. Instead of surmounting their loss, they have developed ways of surviving in a milieu in which the emotional and intellectual challenges have been drastically reduced. Rather than stages, neuroscience now envisions the triune structure —as well as the popular right-brain left-brain opposition— to be constantly interacting, in a constant interplay of one structure with the other, memory and emotion, thought and action, right, left, front, back and center. The reptilian, the mammalian and the human are always interacting, each reaction being adapted to a different kind of situation. Another consequence of this constant interplay is that all activity in the brain happens in a network. For example, it is incorrect to assume that in a situation of heartbreak, one of our three brains is reacting in its specific way, while the other two brains sit back and watch. Although one particular reaction may be dominant, or quicker, it remains that the brain activity always is the product of all three levels of structure. Most interestingly for our purpose, "education can influence which focus dominates." (Caine et al. 1990)

If one takes into account the updating of the triune brain theory, it remains a superb pedagogical device to enter a conversation that has been going on for the last thirty years. As Jaak Panksepp (2004) writes : "This three-layered conceptualization helps us grasp the overall function of higher brain areas better than any other scheme yet devised. Of course, exceptions can be found to all generalizations, and it must be kept in mind that the brain is a massively interconnected organ whose every part can find an access pathway to any other part. Even though many specialists have criticized the overall accuracy of the image of a 'triune brain', the conceptualization provides a useful overview of mammalian brain organization above the lower brain stem. [...] Paul MacLean's triune brain concept is supported by a variety of observations. Although a debatable simplification from a strictly neuroanatomical perspective, MacLean's formulation provides a clear and straightforward way to begin conceptualizing the brain's overall organization."

A number of experts among who are Konner, (1991) and McKinney, (2000) have recognized that the three layers of the brain and their associated behavioral complexes do exist in the brain, although, again, specialized research now uses more detailed maps than this rough division of the brain in three layers of evolution. Today, those who refer to MacLean's theory use it not so much to discuss where the human brain falls on the scale of evolutionary progress, but rather to discover which selective forces in the culture can shape it.

BIBLIOGRAPHY

Association. (1994). *Diagnostic and statistical manual of mental disorders: DSM-IV.* (4th ed.). Washington, DC: American Psychiatric Association.

Bachelard, G. (1946). *La terre et les rêveries du repos.* Paris, France: Corti.

Bachelard, G. (1971). *The poetics of reverie.* (D. Russell, Trans.). Boston, MA: Beacon Press (Original work published 1960).

Bachelard, G. (2005). *Earth and reveries of repose: An essay on images of interiority.* (M. Jones, Trans.). Dallas, TX: Dallas Institute of Humanities & Culture.

Badenoch, B. (2008). *Being a brain-wise therapist: a practical guide to interpersonal neurobiology.* New York, NY: Norton.

Beebe, B. (2004). Faces in Relation: A Case Study. *Psychoanalytic Dialogues, 14*(1), 1-51. doi:10.1080/10481881409348771

Beebe, B. (2007). Preface. In L. Carli & C. Rodini (Eds.), *On intersubjective theories: The implicit and the*

257

explicit in interpersonal relations. Retrieved from http://
nyspi.org/Communication_Sciences/PDF/Infant%20
research%20and%20adult%20treatment/BB%20
2008%20Intersubjective%20theories%20Rodini%20
preface.pdf

Bekoff, M. (2007). The emotional lives of animals: a leading
scientist explores animal joy, sorrow, and empathy and
why they matter. Novato, CA: New World Library.

Bloom, H. (2000). *How to read and why.* New York, NY:
Scribner.

Bonnano, G. (2009) *The Other Side of Sadness: What the
New Science of Bereavement Tells Us About Life After
Loss.* New York, NY: Basic Books.

Borofka, D. (2009). *Memory, muses, memoir.* New York,
NY: iUniverse.

Bosnak, R. (2007) *Embodiment: Creative Imagination in
Medicine, Art and Travel.* New York, NY: Routledge.

Bowlby, J. (1980). *Loss: Sadness and depression.* London,
England: Hogarth Press.

Bradshaw, G. A., & Schore, A. N. (2007). How elephants
are opening doors: Developmental neuroethology,
attachment and social context. *Ethology, 113*(5), 426-
436. doi:10.1111/j.1439-0310.2007.01333.x

Brown, T. (2003). *Making truth: metaphor in science.*
Chicago, IL: University of Illinois press.

Bruner, J. (1990). *Acts of meaning: four lectures on mind and culture*. Cambridge, MA: Harvard University Press.

Butler, A. B. and Hodos, W. (2005). *Comparative Vertebrate Neuroanatomy: Evolution and Adaptation*, 2nd Edition. New York, NY: John Wiley & Sons..

Byrne, R. (2006). *The secret*. London, England: Simon & Schuster.

Cabot, C. R., & Reid, J. C. (2001). *Jung, my mother and I: the analytic diaries of Catharine Rush Cabot*. Einsiedeln, Switzerland: Daimon.

Caine, R. N., and Caine, G. (1990). *Making Connections: Teaching and the Human Brain*. Nashville, TN: Incentive Publications.

Cambray, J. (2002). Synchronicity and emergence. *American Imago, 59*(4), 409-434. doi:10.1353/aim.2002.0023

Cambray, J. (2004). *Analytical psychology: Contemporary perspectives on Jungian analysis*. New York, NY: Brunner-Routledge.

Chua, A., (2011). *The Battle Hymn of the Tiger Mother*. London, England: Bloomsbury Press

Chugani, H. T., Behen, M. E., Muzik, O., Juhász, C., Nagy, F., & Chugani, D. C. (2001). Local brain functional activity following early deprivation: A study of postinstitutionalized Romanian orphans. *NeuroImage, 14*(6), 1290-1301. doi:10.1006/nimg.2001.0917

Comte-Sponville, A. (2002). *Traité du Désespoir et de la Béatitude*. Paris, France: Éditions Quadrige.

Conforti, M. (2003). Field, Form and Fate: Patterns in mind, nature, and psyche. New Orleans, LA: Spring Journal Books.

Cozolino, L. (2002). *The neuroscience of psychotherapy: building and rebuilding the human brain*. New York, NY: Norton.

Cozolino, L. (2006). *The neuroscience of human relationships: attachment and the developing social brain*. New York, NY: Norton.

Crittenden, P. M., & Landini, A. (2011) *The Adult Attachment Interview: Assessing Psychological and Interpersonal Strategies*. New York, N.Y

Cyrulnik, B. (2007). *Talking of love on the edge of a precipice*. London, England: Allen Lane.

Cyrulnik, B. (2009). *Resilience: how your inner strength can set you free from the past*. London, England: Penguin Books.

Damasio, A. (1994). *Descartes' error: emotion, reason, and the human brain*. New York, NY: Putnam.

Damasio, A. (2003). *Looking for Spinoza: joy, sorrow, and the human brain*. New York, NY: Harcourt.

Deacon, T. (1997). *The symbolic species: the co-evolution of language and the brain.* New York, NY: Norton.

Downing, C. (1991). *Mirrors of the self: archetypal images that shape your life.* New York, NY: Tarcher.

Ehrenreich, B. (2009). *Bright-sided: how the relentless promotion of positive thinking has undermined America.* New York, NY: Metropolitan Books.

Fonagy, P., Steele, H., & Steele, M. (1991). Maternal representations of attachment during pregnancy predict the organization of infant-mother attachment at one year of age. *Child Development, 62*(5), 891. doi:10.1111/1467-8624.ep9112161635

Fonagy, P., Gergely, G., Jurist, E. L., & Target, M. (2002). *Affect regulation, mentalization, and the development of the self.* London, England: Karnac.

Fonagy, P., & Target, M. (2008). Attachment, trauma, and psychoanalysis: Where psychoanalysis meets neuroscience. In E. L. Jurist, A. Slade, & S. Bergner (Eds.), *Mind to mind: Infant research, neuroscience, and psychoanalysis.* (pp. 15-49). New York, NY: Other Press.

Gazzaniga, M. (1998). *The mind's past.* Berkeley, CA University of California Press.

Gerhardt, S. (2004). *Why love matters: how affection shapes a baby's brain.* New York, NY: Brunner-Routledge.

Gilbert, D. T. (2006). *Stumbling on happiness.* New York, N.Y: Knopf.

Glenn, D. (2009). A teaching experiment shows students how to grasp big concepts. *Chronicle of Higher Education, 56*(13), A1-A10.

Goodwin, D. (1994). *No ordinary time: Franklin and Eleanor Roosevelt: the home front in World War II.* New York, NY: Simon & Schuster.

Goleman, D. (1996). *Emotional intelligence: why it can matter more than IQ.* London, England: Bloomsbury Press.

Gould, S. (2007). *Punctuated equilibrium.* Cambridge, MA: Harvard University Press.

Guggenbühl, A. (2009). Love: Our most cherished anarchist, or path to failure? In N. Riain, S. Wirth, & J. Hill (Eds.), *Intimacy: Venturing the uncertainties of the heart* (pp. 141-152). New Orleans, LA: Spring Journal Books.

Harrison, R. (2008). *Gardens: an essay on the human condition.* Chicago, IL: University of Chicago Press.

Hawthorne, N. (1850). *The scarlet letter: a romance.* Boston, MA: Ticknor Reed and Fields.

Hennighausen, K., & Lyons-Ruth, K. (2010). Disorganization of attachment strategies in infancy and childhood. In R. Tremblay, R. Barr, R. Peters, & M. Boivin (Eds.), *Encyclopedia on early childhood development* (pp. 1-7). Montreal, Quebec, Canada: Centre of Excellence for Early Childhood Development.

Retrieved from http://www.child-encyclopedia.com/ documents/Hennighausen-LyonsRuthANGxp_rev.pdf

Hesse, E., & Main, M. (2000). Disorganized infant, child, and adult attachment: Collapse in behavioral and attentional strategies. *Journal of the American Psychoanalytic Association, 48*(4), 1097-1127. doi:10.1177/00030651000480041101

Hillman, J. (1964). *Suicide and the soul.* New York, NY: Harper & Row.

Hillman. J. (1972). *Pan and the Nightmare.* New York, N.Y: Spring Publications.

Hillman, J. (1975a). *Loose ends: primary papers in archetypal psychology.* Dallas, TX: Spring.

Hillman, J. (1975b). *Re-visioning psychology.* New York, NY: Harper & Row.

Hillman, J. (Ed.). (1979). *Puer papers.* Irving, TX: Spring.

Hillman, J. (1989). From mirror to window: Curing psychoanalysis of its narcissism. *Spring Journal, 49,* 62-75.

Hillman, J. (2010). *Alchemical psychology.* Putnam, CT: Spring.

Hofer, M. A. (1995). An evolutionary perspective on anxiety. In S. P. Roose & R. A. Glick (Eds.), *Anxiety as symptom and signal* (pp. 17-38). Hillsdale, NJ: Analytic Press.

Hofer, M. A., & Sullivan, R. M. (2008). Toward a neurobiology of attachment. In C. A. Nelson & M. Luciana (Eds.), *Handbook of developmental cognitive neuroscience* (2nd ed., pp. 787-805). Cambridge, MA: MIT Press.

Hogenson, G. B. (2001). The Baldwin effect: A neglected influence on C. G. Jung's evolutionary thinking. *Journal of Analytical Psychology, 46*(4), 591-611. doi:10.1111/1465-5922.00269

Holmes, J. (1996). *Attachment, intimacy, autonomy: using attachment theory in adult psychotherapy.* Northvale, NJ: Jason Aronson.

Horney, K. (1939). *New ways in psychoanalysis.* New York, NY: Norton.

Horowitz, M. J., Siegel, B., Holen, A., Bonanno, G. A., Milbrath, C., & Stinson, C. H. (2003). Diagnostic criteria for complicated grief disorder. *Focus, 1*(3), 290-298.

Hutterer, J., & Liss, M. (2006). Cognitive development, memory, trauma, treatment: An integration of psychoanalytic and behavioral concepts in light of current neuroscience research. *Journal of the American Academy of Psychoanalysis & Dynamic Psychiatry, 34*(2), 287-302. doi:10.1521/jaap.2006.34.2.287

Insel, T.R., & Numan, M. (2011) *The Neurobiology of Maternal Behavior* . New York, NY: Springer (in press)

Jacobs, W. J. (1983). *Eleanor Roosevelt: A Life of Happiness and Tears*. New York: Coward-McCann.

Jung, C. G. (1967). Symbols of transformation. In H. Read, M. Fordham, G. Adler, & W. McGuire (Eds.), F. C. Hull (Trans.), *The collected works of C. G. Jung* (Vol. 5). Princeton, NJ: Princeton University Press (Original work published 1912).

Kalsched, D. (1996). *The inner world of trauma: archetypal defenses of the personal spirit*. New York, NY: Routledge.

Kandel, E (1998). *A New Intellectual Framework for Psychiatry?* American J. Psychiatry, 1998, 155, p 460.

Kearney, M. (2000). *A place of healing: working with suffering in living and dying*. New York, NY: Oxford University Press.

Kohut, H. (1966). Forms and transformations of narcissism. *Journal of the American Psychoanalytic Association*, *14*(2), 243-272. doi:10.1177/000306516601400201

Kohut, H. (1971). *The analysis of the self : a systematic approach to the psychoanalytic treatment of narcissistic personality disorders*. New York, NY: International Universities Press.

Konigsberg. R. D., (2011). *The truth about Grief.* New York, N.Y: Simon &Schuster.

Konner, M. (1991). Childhood. New York, NY: Little Brown.

Knox, J. (2003*). Archetype, attachment, analysis: Jungian psychology and the emergent mind.* New York, NY: Brunner-Routledge.

Lasch, C. (1979). *The culture of narcissism: American life in an age of diminishing expectations.* New York, NY: Warner.

Lane, R. D. (2008). Neural substrates of implicit and explicit emotional processes: A unifying framework for psychosomatic medicine. *Psychosomatic Medicine, 70*(2), 214-231. doi:10.1097/PSY.0b013e3181647e44

LeDoux, J. (1996). *The emotional brain: the mysterious underpinnings of emotional life.* New York, NY: Simon & Schuster.

LeDoux, J. (2002). *Synaptic self: How our brains become who we are.* New York, NY: Penguin.

Lewis, T., Amini, F., & Lannon, R. (2000). *A general theory of love.* New York, NY: Random House.

Long, E. (2009). Metaphor, personification & anthromorphization in contemporary popular media representations of science (Unpublished Doctoral Dissertation). Pacifica Graduate Institute, Carpinteria, CA.

Lynch, J. (1977). *The broken heart: the medical consequences of loneliness.* New York, NY: Basic Books.

Lyons-Ruth, K. (1998). Implicit relational knowing: Its role in development and psychoanalytic treatment.

Infant Mental Health Journal, 19(3), 282-289. doi:10.1002/(SICI)1097-0355(199823)19:3<282::AID-IMHJ3>3.0.CO;2-O

Lyons-Ruth, K. (1999). The two-person unconscious: Intersubjective dialogue, enactive relational representation, and the emergence of new forms of relational organization. *Psychoanalytic Inquiry, 19*(4), 576-617. doi:10.1080/07351699909534267

Mahaffey, P. (2005). Jung's depth psychology and yoga sadhana. In K. Jacobsen (Ed.), *Theory and practice of yoga: Essays in honour of Gerald James Larson* (pp. 385-408). Leiden, The Netherlands: Brill.

Mancia, M. (2006). Implicit memory and early unrepressed unconscious: Their role in the therapeutic process (How the neurosciences can contribute to psychoanalysis). *International Journal of Psycho-Analysis, 87*(1), 83-103.

Mar, R. A. (2004). The neuropsychology of narrative: Story comprehension, story production and their interrelation. *Neuropsychologia, 42*(10), 1414-1434. doi:10.1016/j.neuropsychologia.2003.12.016

Marlan, S. (2005). *The black sun: the alchemy and art of darkness*. College Station: Texas A & M University Press.

Masterson, J. (1993). *The emerging self: a developmental, self, and object relations approach to the treatment of the closet narcissistic disorder of the self.* New York, NY: Brunner/Mazel.

Melville, H. (1851). *Moby-Dick or, The whale.* New York, NY: Harper.

Michaux, H. (1963). *Passages 1937-1963.* Nouvelle édition revue et augmentée. Paris, France: Gallimard.

Miller, A. (1981). *The drama of the gifted child.* New York, NY: Basic Books.

Miller, D. (1995). Nothing almost sees miracles! Self and no-Self in psychology and religion. *Journal of the Psychology of Religion, 4-5,* 1-26.

Miller, D. (2005). *Three faces of God: traces of the Trinity in literature and life* (New ed.). New Orleans, LA: Spring Journal Books (Original work published 1986).

Millon, T. (2004). *Personality disorders in modern life* (2nd ed.). Hoboken, NJ: Wiley.

Modell, A. H. (1997). The synergy of memory, affects and metaphor. *Journal of Analytical Psychology, 42*(1), 105-117.

Murdock, M. (2003). *Unreliable truth: on memoir and memory.* New York, NY: Seal Press.

Offer, M. (1995). An evolutionary perspective on anxiety. In S. Roose (Ed.), *Anxiety as symptom and signal* (pp. 25-27). Hillsdale, NJ: Analytic Press.

Panksepp, J. (1998). *Affective neuroscience: the foundations of human and animal emotions*. New York, NY: Oxford University Press.

Panksepp, J. (2003). At the interface of the affective, behavioral, and cognitive neurosciences: Decoding the emotional feelings of the brain. *Brain and Cognition, 52*(1), 4-14. doi:10.1016/S0278-2626(03)00003-4

Panksepp, J., (Ed.) (2004) *A Textbook of Biological Psychiatry*, New York, NY: John Wiley & Sons

Panksepp, J. (2008). The power of the word may reside in the power of affect. *Integrative Psychological & Behavioral Science, 42*(1), 47-55. doi:10.1007/s12124-007-9036-5

Pearson, C. (1986). *The hero within: six archetypes we live by*. San Francisco, CA: Harper & Row.

Phillips, A. (1994). *On flirtation*. Cambridge, MA: Harvard University Press.

Phillips, A. (2005). *Going sane: maps of happiness*. New York, NY: HarperCollins.

Prins, A., Kaloupek, D. G., & Keane, T. M. (1995). Psychophysiological evidence for autonomic arousal and startle in traumatized adult populations. In M. J. Friedman, D. S. Charney, & A. Y. Deutch (Eds.), *Neurobiological and clinical consequences of stress: From normal adaptation to post-traumatic stress disorder*. (pp. 291-314). Philadelphia, PA: Lippincott Williams & Wilkins.

Proust, M. (1996). *La fin de la jalousie: Et autres nouvelles*. Paris, France: Gallimard. (Original work published 1923)

Proust, M. (1954). *A la recherche du temps perdu*. Paris, France: Gallimard.

Proust, M. (1990). *Le temps retrouvé*. Paris, France: Gallimard. (Original work published 1927)

Ratey, J. J. (2002). *A user's guide to the brain: Perception, attention and the four theaters of the brain*. New York, NY: Vintage Books.

Roose, S. (1995). *Anxiety as symptom and signal*. Hillsdale, NJ: Analytic Press.

Rossi, E. L. (2007). *The breakout heuristic: The neuroscience of mirror neurons, consciousness and human creativity*. Phoenix, AZ: The Milton Erickson Foundation Press.

Rowland, S. (2002). *Jung: a feminist revision*. Malden, MA: Blackwell.

Rowland, S. (2005). *Jung as a writer*. New York, NY: Routledge.

Russell. F., (1993) *Eleanor Roosevelt: A Life of Discovery*. New York: Clarion Books.

Sander, L. (1977). The regulation of exchange in the infant caretaker system and some aspects of the context-content relationship. In M. Lewis & L. Rosenblum (Eds.), *Interaction, conversation, and the development of language* (pp. 133-156). New York, NY: Wiley.

Sander, L. W. (2002). Thinking differently: Principles of process in living systems and the specificity of being known. Psychoanalytic *Dialogues, 12*(1), 11-42. doi:10.1080/10481881209348652

Schoen, D. (2009). *The war of the gods in addiction: C.G. Jung, Alcoholics Anonymous, and archetypal evil.* New Orleans, LA: Spring Journal Books.

Schwartz-Salant, N. (2007). *The black nightgown: the fusional complex and the unlived life.* Wilmette, IL: Chiron.

Schore, A. N. (2002). Dysregulation of the right brain: a fundamental mechanism of traumatic attachment and the psychopathogenesis of posttraumatic stress disorder. *Australian and New Zealand Journal of Psychiatry, 36*(1), 9-30. doi:10.1046/j.1440-1614.2002.00996.x

Schore, A. (2003). *Affect regulation and the repair of the self.* New York, NY: Norton.

Schore, A. (2003b). *Affect dysregulation and disorders of the self.* New York, NY: Norton.

Shore, A. (2008). Paradigm shift: The right brain and the relational unconscious. *Psychologist-Psychoanalyst, 28*(3), 20–25.

Schore, J. R., & Schore, A. N. (2008). Modern attachment theory: The central role of affect regulation in development and treatment. *Clinical Social Work Journal, 36*(1), 9-20. doi:10.1007/s10615-007-0111-7

Sharp, D. (1991). *Jung lexicon: a primer of terms and concepts.* Toronto, Canada: Inner City Books.

Siegel, D. (1999). *The developing mind: toward a neurobiology of interpersonal experience.* New York, NY: Guilford Press.

Siegel, D. (2003). *Healing Trauma: Attachment, Mind, Body and Brain.* New York: Norton. Co-edited with Marion Solomon.

Siegel, D. (2007). *The Mindful-Brain-in-Psychotherapy/ The Mindful Brain: Reflection and Attunement in the Cultivation of Well-Being.* New York, NY: Norton.

Siegel, D. (2009). *The Healing Power of Emotion: Affective Neuroscience, Development & Clinical Practice.* New York, NY: Norton.

Siegel, D. (2010) *The-Mindful-Therapist/ The Mindful Therapist: A Clinician's Guide to Mindsight and Neural Integration.* New York, NY: Norton.

Solms, M. (2002). *The brain and the inner world: an introduction to the neuroscience of subjective experience.* New York, NY: Other Press.

Solomon, M. (2003). *Healing trauma: attachment, mind, body, and brain.* New York, NY: Norton.

Somerville, M. (1996). *Eleanor Roosevelt As I Knew Her.* McLean, VA: EPM Publications.

Spiegel, J., Severino, S. K., & Morrison, N. K. (2000). The role of attachment functions in psychotherapy. *Journal of Psychotherapy Practice & Research, 9*(1), 25-32.

Stark, M. (1999). *Modes of Therapeutic Action.* Jason Aronson. New Jersey: Northvale.

Stein, M. (1998). *Jung's map of the soul: an introduction.* Chicago, IL: Open Court.

Stein, M. (2006). Individuation. In R. K. Papadopoulos (Ed.), *The handbook of Jungian psychology: Theory, practice and applications.* (pp. 196-214). New York, NY: Routledge.

Stern, D., Sander, L., Nahum, J., Harrison, A., Lyons-Ruth, K., Morgan, A., Bruschweilerstern, N., et al. (1998). Non-interpretive mechanisms in psychoanalytic therapy: The 'something more' than interpretation. *The International Journal of Psychoanalysis, 79*(5), 903-921.

Stern, D. (2004). *The present moment in psychotherapy and everyday life.* New York, NY: Norton.

Stewart, C. (2008). *Dire emotions and lethal behaviors: eclipse of the life instinct.* New York, NY: Routledge.

Tacy, D. (2004). *The Spirituality Revolution: The Emergence of contemporary Spirituality.* New York, NY: Routledge.

Taylor, J. (2006). *My stroke of insight: a brain scientist's personal journey*. New York, NY: Viking.

Taylor, S. E., Klein, L. C., Lewis, B. P., Gruenewald, T. L., Gurung, R. A. R., & Updegraff, J. A. (2000). Biobehavioral responses to stress in females: Tend-and-befriend, not fight-or-flight. *Psychological Review, 107*(3), 411-429. doi:10.1037/0033-295X.107.3.411

Tronick, E. (2007). *The neurobehavioral and social-emotional development of infants and children*. New York, NY: Norton.

Tulving, E. (2000). *The Oxford handbook of memory*. New York, NY: Oxford University Press.

Turbayne, C. (1971). *The myth of metaphor* (Rev. ed.). Columbia: University of South Carolina Press.

Twenge, J., & Campbell, W. K. (2009). *The narcissism epidemic: living in the age of entitlement*. New York, NY: Free Press.

Verplaetse, J., Braeckman, J., De Schrijver, J., & Vanneste, S. (Eds.). (2009). *The moral brain: essays on the evolutionary and neuroscientific aspects of morality*. New York, NY: Springer.

Youngs, J.W., (2000). *Eleanor Roosevelt: A Personal and Public Life*. Edited by Oscar Handlin. Boston: Little, Brown, 1985. Reprint, New York: Longman

Watt, D. F. (2004). Psychotherapy in an age of neuroscience. In J. Corrigall & H. Wilkinson (Eds.), *Revolutionary connections: Psychotherapy and neuroscience* (pp. 79-115). New York, NY: Karnac.

Watt, D. F. (2005). Social bonds and the nature of empathy. *Journal of Consciousness Studies, Emotion experience, 12*(8-10), 185-209.

Wilkinson, M. (2003). Undoing trauma: Contemporary neuroscience. A Jungian clinical perspective. *Journal of Analytical Psychology, 48*(2), 235-253.

Wilkinson, M. (2004). The mind-brain relationship: The emergent self. *Journal of Analytical Psychology, 49*(1), 83-101. doi:10.1111/j.0021-8774.2004.0442.x

Wilkinson, M. (2006). *Coming into mind: The main-brain relationship: A Jungian clinical perspective.* London, England: Routledge.

Wilkinson, M. (2007a). Jung and neuroscience: The making of mind. In A. Casement (Ed.), *Who owns Jung?* (pp. 339-362). London England: Karnac Books.

Wilkinson, M. (2007b). Coming into mind: Contemporary neuroscience, attachment, and the psychological therapies: A clinical perspective. *Attachment: New directions in psychotherapy and relational psychoanalysis, 1*(3), 323-330.

Wilkinson, M. (2010). *Changing minds in therapy: emotion, attachment, trauma, and neurobiology.* New York, NY: Norton.

Wilson, E. O. (1998). Consilience: The unity of knowledge. New York, NY: Knopf.

Young, K., & Saver, J. L. (2001). The Neurology of Narrative. *SubStance, 30*(1), 72-84. doi:10.1353/sub.2001.0020

Zweig C., & Wolf, S., (1997) *Romancing the Shadow.* Ballantine, N.Y.

Zoja, L. (2010). Carl Gustav Jung as a historical-cultural phenomenon. *International Journal of Jungian Studies.* Vol.2,No.2, September 2010, 141-150

ENDNOTES

1. Carmina Burana (*Song of Beuren*) is a collection of twelfth and thirteenth-century poems written by defrocked monks who had freed themselves of monastic discipline, joining students and wandering minstrels. The poems describe the beauty of spring and of new love, the exuberance of tavern life and the indulgence of gluttony and drink, sexual passion, fear of death and the shortness of life.

2. The lyrics were written by D. Hall and P. Hampton and made famous by the interpreter Johnny Cash, and later by his daughter, Roseanne Cash.

3. Proust (1996). My translation.

4. Solms (2002).

5. "Bereavement is generally diagnosed instead of Adjustment Disorder when the reaction is an expectable response to the death of a loved one. The diagnosis of Adjustment Disorder may be appropriate when the reaction is in excess of, or more prolonged than, what

would be expected." American Psychiatric Association (1994, p. 682).

6. Horowitz et al. (2003, p. 298).

7. Martha Stark (1999), calls this "relentless hope" and links it, like most therapists do, to the failure to mourn. As for the French philosopher Andre Comte-Sponville (2002) he writes beautifully about the danger of living with the wrong kind of hope. He wrote a *Treatise on Despair and Bliss!* (*Traité du Désespoir et de la Béatitude.*)

8. What Jung called the *teleological aspect of the psyche*, as if it had a plan for us to move beyond mom, dad and the past traumas, to express our unique gifts. See Stein (1998).

9. "Quant au bonheur, il n'a presque qu'une seule utilité, rendre le malheur possible. Il faut que dans le bonheur nous formions des liens bien doux et bien forts de confiance et d'attachement pour que leur rupture nous cause le déchirement si précieux qui s'appelle le malheur. Si l'on n'avait pas été heureux, ne fût-ce que par l'espérance, les malheurs seraient sans cruauté et par conséquent sans fruit." Proust (1990, p. 907). My translation.

10. Hillman (1975, p. 66).

11. In order to avoid too much of a technical discussion, an «updating» of MacLean's theory is the object of a short addendum at the end of this book.

12. In James Hillman (1975b, p. 12) terms: « So we shall not use the terms anthropomorphism and animism but rather the term personifying to signify the basic psychological activity—the spontaneous experiencing, envisioning and speaking of the configurations of existence as psychic presences—and hopefully thereby save this authentic activity from being condemned as personification.»

13. The work of Joseph Ledoux clarified the function of the amygdala in stocking our memories; he demonstrated how, along with the amygdala's central role, the whole brain is involved. LeDoux (1996 and 2002).

14. Taylor (2006, p. 18).

15. See: Offer (1995, pp. 25-27). See also Fonagy @al. (2008), Cambray (2004) and Cyrulnik (2009).

16. See: Bekoff (2007).

17. See: Lynch (1977).

18. Researchers at The Sackler Institute for Developmental Psychobiology at the Columbia University College of Physicians and Surgeons have developed ways

of appraising how, in laboratory rats, early maternal separation affects the offspring's vulnerability to disease. They have confirmed many of the regulatory processes that were at the level of hypothesis in psychological theories of attachment. Their research offers a neurological basis for understanding the damage that results from a traumatic separation from the usual caregivers or partners, and the impact it has at the molecular, cellular, behavioral, and psychological levels.

19. See Kearney (2000), who describes the healing temples in Ancient Greece. Cleansing the patient of his/her miasma was a synonym for healing.

20. Lewis, Amini, & Lannon (2000, p. 79).

21. See: Beebee (2008), Tronick (2007), Stern & al, (1988) See also Ainsworth (1979). See also *The Adult Attachment Interview* developed by Kaplan & Main, to be published in 2011, in Crittendon (2011).

22. See Kalched (1996).

23. This one from Elvis!

24. See Knox (2003).

25. See James Hillman's chapter on Masturbation *in Pan and the Nightmare*. He concludes the chapter with

this thought: "Because it is the only sexual activity performed alone, we may not judge it solely in terms of its service to the species or to society. Rather than focusing upon its useless role in external civilization and procreation, we may reflect upon its usefulness for internal culture and creativity. By intensifying interiority with joy—and with conflict and shame, and by vivifying fantasy, masturbation, which has no purpose for species or society, yet brings genital pleasure, fantasy and guilt to the individual as psychic subject. It sexualizes fantasy, brings body to mind, intensifies the experience of conscience and confirms the powerful reality of the introverted psyche—was it not invented for the solitary shepherd piping through the empty places of our inscapes and who re-appears when we are thrown into solitude. By constellating Pan, masturbation brings nature and its complexity back into the opus contra naturam of soul-making."

26. Taylor et al. (2000).

27. Cambray, J., and Carter, L., (2004) .

28. Phillips (1994, p. 17).

29. Lewis, Amini, & Lannon (2000, p. 33).

30. See Fonagy (2002).

31. Many therapeutic approaches now explicitly refer to the

neurological dimension of emotional change, offering methods and approaches that claim to train the brain to reduce psychological stress, anxiety and depression. No one approach can claim a copyright on the healing process of the brain, but I find it interesting that all these approaches are based on the same conditions that facilitate neurogenesis.

32. It is especially dangerous in cultures such as ours, where the star system offers ready made models of "the good life".

33. I hope that Rhonda Byrne's bestseller, *The Secret* (2006), will go down in history as an example of a terrible confusion between science and faith. Like all teachings from pseudo gurus who want you to believe in magical thinking, it suggests that it is enough to send out messages to the universe to come rescue you, and to think positively. This young woman was helped by reading Connie Zweig (1997) : *Romancing the Shadow*, which explain, in non-jargon language, the Jungian notion of shadow and offers simple exercises to get acquainted with one's destructive shadow

34. "Une bonne étude des souffrances équilibrantes n'a pas été faite, que je sache. Il y a pourtant déjà quelque temps que l'humanité souffre. Pour les souffrances morales, il y a un peu plus d'instructions dans ce sens ! Quoiqu'il y ait des sots qui cherchent à un malheur le

contrepoids non d'un autre malheur, mais du bonheur!"
Michaux (1963, p. 123). My translation.

35. Daniel Gilbert's (2006) study of the neurological factor
    that enhance happiness is a convincing demonstration of
    the power of a positive outlook on life.

36. Ernest Lawrence Rossi's latest book (2007) summarizes
    many years of study of the function of dreams as a
    precursor to psychic growth, emphasizing the role of
    Milton Erickson in psychotherapy and hypnosis. Before
    now, much of it could only be obtained by gathering
    it from various and diverse sources. Rossi bridges the
    gap between Jungian psychotherapy and Ericksonian
    approaches to hypnosis.

37. Kübler-Ross. E., (1969).

38. See Konigsberg. R. D., (2011).

39. See Bonnano's (2004).

40. Bachelard (2010, p. 44).

41. Miller (1986/2005).

42. Jerome Bruner was a professor of psychology at
    Harvard (1952-72) and then at Oxford (1972-80)
    as well as at the New School for Social Research in
    New York City. He served on the President's Science

Advisory Committee during the Kennedy and Johnson administrations.

43. Bruner (1990).

44. Bloom (2000, p. 183).

45. "We do not, however, have to get rid of ourselves in order to rid ourselves of the idea [of suicide]. Rather than seeing it through to our end, we can see through it to *its* end." Hillman 2006. p 125.

46. Michael Gazzaniga is director of the Center for Cognitive Neuroscience at Dartmouth College and the author of *The Mind's Past* (1998).

47. The group leader used the following three resources on memoir writing: Maureen Murdock: *Unreliable Truth: on Memoir and Memory* (2003). Chris Downing: *Mirrors of the Self: Archetypal Images Shape Your Life* (1991). Deb Borofka: *Memory, Muses, Memoir* (2009).

48. See: Long (2009).

49. Brown (2003, p. 126).

50. Turbayne (1971, p. 22).

51. Some authors offer a map of a map, as for example does Murray Stein in *Jung's Map of the Soul* (1998). Stein writes in his Introduction: '[Jung's] theory is the

284

map he created to communicate his understanding of the psyche. So it is Jung's map of the soul that I will attempt to describe in this book by leading you, the reader, into and through the territory of his writings. In doing so, I am presenting a map of a map [....]' (p. 3).

52. 'What aspects of human social organization and adaptation wouldn't benefit from the evolution of language?' asks Terrence Deacon, a biological anthropologist at the University of California, Berkeley, in *The Symbolic Species: The Coevolution of Language and the Brain* (1997, p. 377).

53. See Bosnak (2007).

54. The actual tendency to cut on literary training in schools has an impact not only on the imagination, but on the psychological ability to relate to others. Without 'good words" to express one's emotions, the brain regresses to lower levels of consciousness.

55. Hillman (1975b, p. 47).

56. "On croit que selon son désir on changera autour de soi les choses, on le croit parce que, hors de là, on ne voit aucune solution favorable. On ne pense pas à celle qui se produit le plus souvent et est favorable aussi: nous n'arrivons pas à changer les choses selon notre désir, mais peu à peu notre désir change. La situation

que nous espérions changer parce qu'elle nous était insupportable nous devient indifférente. Nous n'avons pas pu surmonter l'obstacle, comme nous le voulions absolument, mais la vie nous l'a fait tourner, dépasser, et c'est à peine alors si en nous retournant vers le lointain du passé nous pouvons l'apercevoir, tant il est devenu imperceptible." (Proust, 1954. p. 451). My translation.

57. Taylor (2006, pp. 120-121).

58. Melville (1851, Chapter 44).

59. American Psychiatric Association (1994).

60. See Cozolino (2006), Fonagy (2002) and (2008).

61. Bowlby (1980).

62. Bachelard (1946, p. 28). My translation.

63. My father was an electrical contractor; my first stack of metaphors to understand the psyche was through metaphors of shorts, overloaded circuits, power failures, power differential, power shortages, shock and electrocution. I was impressed by the beautiful complexity of blueprints showing the inner wiring of a big building such as a school or a hospital and equally impressed by my father's uncanny ability to figure out, better than any engineer on site, any mistake in a

blueprint. Seeing him at work was my first exposure to the glory of rational thinking. He is one of my welcome ghosts, a provider of metaphors. My repertoire has since expanded: the whole sensate reality is a repertoire of metaphors to pick and choose from.

64. Marlan (2005, p. 2).

65. Jung (1967, p. 357).

66. "The retrieval of episodic information […] is not merely an objective account of what has happened or what has been seen or heard. Its contents are infused with the idiosyncratic perspectives, emotions, and thoughts of the person doing the remembering. It necessarily involves the feeling that the present recollection is a re-experience of something that has happened before. … '[…] The author also mentions how the act of recollecting and reflecting upon one's past is cognitively and neurologically similar to the act of anticipating one's future, although we don't use the word memory in that case. (p.598) By contrast to the autonetic memory, a noetic (knowing) memory is one where we don't need to recall or relive the past to remember something that has become a routine, like reaching for your wallet in the back pocket." Tulving (2000).

67. Tulving (2000, p. 598).

HEARTBREAK

68. Prasad (2007). See also information on "broken heart syndrome" as well as "cardiomyopathy" offered on the website of the Division of Cardiovascular Diseases and Department of Internal Medicine, Mayo Clinic and Mayo Foundation. http://www.mayoclinic.com/

69. For more information, see also the website: http://www.hopkinsmedicine.org/asc/

70. James Hillman (1975b) developed this psychological concept of "seeing through" in his seminal work: *Re-Visioning Psychology*. He defines consciousness as a "seeing through" to the myth, the symbol, the emotion, the complex... one is possessed by.

71. Luigi Zoja (2010) says it with elegance: " Complexes and neuroses cannot be addressed only as individual problems. The individual not only originates in society and withing a culture but is awyas in relation to them. Therefore the medical model of he natural sciences is not sufficient. [...]. In this sense, Jung has left an unresolved antinomy. On the one hand, he says that the origin of every problem within society can be found in the psyche of the individual. On the other hand, he asserts that the individual psyche is the product of a difficult and intricate differentiation from the collective psyche: even in the original natural state, psyche is still immersed in the collective. Perhaps more than an antinomy, here again we are dealing with a circular

process. The collective psyche is he *historic* origin of the individual one. This latter, however, exactly because it is differentiated, is in turn the *moral* origin of the new collective problems."

72. Stewart (2008).

73. Nietzsche, F. Twilight if the Idols and the Antechrist.

74. Lewis, Gibson, & Lannon (2000)

75. Jane Cabot Reid's book, Jung, My Mother and I (2001), gives a precise sense of the life of the therapeutic community in Zurich at the height of Jung's fame. Most of what was then felt as natural, such as Jung discussing a patient's social background and symptoms with another patient, or the social activities involving the whole analytical community of patients and therapists would be today against the code of ethics of our profession.

76. Patrick Mahaffey (2005, p. 385), a friend and colleague who teaches Hinduism and Buddhism at the Pacifica Graduate Institute in California, writes this : "C.G. Jung regarded yoga to be one of the greatest things the human mind has ever created but believed that the spiritual development in the West has been along entirely different lines. He felt that the West would gradually develop its own yoga. While [my] essay

argues that Jung's belief that yoga is not suitable for Westerners is mistaken, it also suggests that his depth psychology is itself a kind of Western yoga."

77. See Schwartz-Salant (2007).

78. See: Verplaetse, Braeckman, De Schrijver, & Vanneste (2009). Although most scientists discredit the idea of a *moral organ* as phrenologists once did, there is new emerging evidence that specific brain processes enabling moral cognition.

79. Jung, in Sharp (1991).

80. See: Schoen (2009).

81. Pacifica Graduate Institute. See: www. pacifica.edu

82. Guggenbühl (2009, p. 151).

83. The American Psychiatric Association (APA) is the organism responsible for the ongoing revision of the DSM. The DSM-5 (they are dropping the roman numeral for the arabic number) is actually being revised by a group of twenty-seven specialists from psychiatry, psychology, clinical care providers and consumer and family advocates.

84. Diamonds too are forever, but the symbolization of a diamond as a token of love is more recent, and not as

universal. It is the result of a fantastically successful advertisement campaign by De Beers Diamonds, in the nineteenth century.

85. For those interested in alchemy as metaphor for psychological processes, see Hillman, (2010) and Marlan (2005).

86. Interestingly, real gold cannot be attacked by a single acid. It takes the combination of two very strong acids (nitric and hydrochloric acids), a solution the alchemists call 'aqua regia', which means royal water, to dissolve gold.

87. Kohut (1971 and 1966).

88. Horney (1939).

89. Masterson (1993).

90. Milton (2004).

91. Twenge & Campbell (2009)

92. Hillman (1989, pp. 62-75).

93. There are no less than 36,000 different credits cards available to a US citizen as compared to 400 in Canada. This number comprises all the major one, like Visa, Master Card or American Express, but we tend to forget that companies like Esso, Home Depot, Sears,

Amazon…all offer their own brand of credit cards. The total of individual credit cards in circulation in the US was 1.3 billion at the end of 2003, U.S. compared to 9 million in France. (The French and the German use mostly debit cards). See regular information about credit card dept in the industry newsletter the Nilson Report. Also: wws.creditcard.com for detailed statistics.

94. Twenge & Campbell (2009*)*. See also Hill, Victor (2005) *Corporate Narcissism in Accounting Firms.* Pengus Books. Australia.

95. Lasch (1979).

96. It might be useful to examine borderline traits as narcissistic traits and vice versa, especially when it comes to the notion of 'lack of empathy'. Although the narcissist has a more stable self-image and less self-destructiveness, both the narcissist and the borderline personality lack empathy for the other.

97. Doris Kearns Goodwin, in *No Ordinary Time* (1994), wrote how, during the depression and World War II, Eleanor traveled throughout the country, busy becoming more the beloved figure she came to be for the whole country.

98. David Miller, a theologian, formulates the idea this way: "The majority of mystical theologies in the

world's religious traditions hold as a spiritual goal precisely the nothingness and emptiness about which those who suffer today complain. The spiritual goal in these religious traditions is spoken of in a rhetoric that suggests that one should not aspire to achieve self-sense, self-hood, or identity, but that one precisely loose these in favor of a sense of no-self." (1995-1996, p. 4)

99. Harrison (2008, p.164).

100. In defense of the archetype of youth, see: Hillman (1979)

101. Rowland (2002).

102. Miller (1981).

103. Chua (2011).

104. See Cyrulnik, Resilience (2009). And also: Talking of Love on the Edge of a Precipice (2007).

105. Pearson (1986).

106. Hawthorne, *The Scarlet Letter* (1850).

107. "Neurons either thrive when connected in circuit with other neurons, or they die when they sit in isolation without stimulation." Taylor (2006, p. 97).

108. In evolutionary biology, this capacity to adapt is called

by Stephen Jay Gould and Niles Eldridge 'punctuated equilibrium' in opposition to Darwin's 'gradualism'. Gould (2007).

109. Panksepp (1998, p. 16).

110. Eleanor Roosevelt wrote several books about her experiences as a shy girl who reluctantly find herseif in the position of first lady herself : *This Is My Story* (1937), *This I Remember* (1950), *On My Own* (1958), and *Tomorrow Is Now* (published posthumously, 1963).

111. There are many biographies of Eleanor Roosevelt, among which are: 1) Russell. F., (1993) Eleanor Roosevelt: *A Life of Discovery*. New York: Clarion Books. 2) Jacobs, W. J. (1983). *Eleanor Roosevelt*: *A Life of Happiness and Tears.* New York: Coward-McCann. 3) : Somerville, M. (1996) . *Eleanor Roosevelt As I Knew Her.* McLean, VA: EPM Publications. 4) Youngs, J.W., (2000). *Eleanor Roosevelt: A Personal and Public Life.* Edited by Oscar Handlin. Boston: Little, Brown, 1985. Reprint, New York: Longman.

112. See Schore (2003, 2003b). Siegel, D. (1999, 2003, 2007, 2009, 2010).

113. Beebe (2007) Fonagy (2008), Sander (1997), Stern (2004), Tronick (2007).

114. See Cambray (2004), Hogenson (2001), Knox (2003).

115. Mark Solms (1998), director of the Center for Neuro-Psychoanalysis at the New York Psychoanalytic Institute, has compared the clinical insights from depth psychology, especially Freudian, with knowledge generated by neurosciences. He calls this field neuro-psychoanalysis and shows how the brain and what psychologists call the *personality* are intrinsically connected. He is one among many doing this work, demonstrating the need for more interdisciplinary approaches.

116. Ratey (2002, p. 17).

117. Wilson (1988 pp.11-12).

118. Myron Hofer, director of the Sackler Institute for Developmental Psychobiology at Columbia University College of Physicians and Surgeons, has studied how early maternal separation and different patterns of mothering exert long-term effects on offspring vulnerability to disease. See : Hofer & Sullivan (2008). Dr. Hofer writes on his webpage: "through an experimental analysis of the psychobiological interactions that enmesh the infant rat and its mother, we have discovered hidden regulatory processes that have become the basis for a new understanding of the early origins of attachment, the dynamics of the

separation response and the shaping of development by that first relationship. Currently I have become interested in theoretical aspects of development as it relates to evolution and in defining principles that can help bridge the gap between developmental processes at the molecular/cellular, behavioral, and psychological levels."

119. "Similarities [between mammalian animals and humans] in cortical interconnectedness diminish markedly as one begins to compare the more complex secondary and tertiary association cortices where perceptions, as well as most cognitive and rational processes, are generated. In short, multimodal association areas of the cortex, where information among an increasing number of areas, similarities between humans and other animals begin to diminish. The speech cortex is the most multimodal of them all, and there humans and other animals have most decisively parted ways." Panksepp (2000, p. 60).

120. The limbic brain, also called the mammalian brain or emotional brain, is the brain we share with all mammals. It responds to a variety of medications that have the same effect on mammals and humans. Most anti-depressants target the regulation of the limbic brain.

121. "We can now conceptualize basic psychological

processes in neurological terms that appeared terminally stuck in unproductive semantic realms only a few years ago. Neuroscientific riches are now so vast that all subfields of psychology must begin to integrate a new and strange landscape into their thinking if they want to stay on the forefront of scientific inquiry. This new knowledge will have great power to affect human welfare, as well as human self-conception. It is finally possible to credibly infer the natural order of the 'inner causes' of behavior, including the emotional process that activate many of the coherent psychobehavioral tendencies animals and humans exhibit spontaneously without much prior learning. These natural brain processes help create the deeply felt value structures that govern much of our behavior, whether learned or unlearned. This new mode of thought is the intellectual force behind affective neuroscience." Panksepp (2000, p. 11).

122. In the words of David Tacey (2004, p. 2): "What is the spirituality revolution? It is a spontaneous movement in society, a new interest in the reality of spirit and its healing effects on life, health community and well-being. [...] The spiritual life is no longer a specialist concern, confined to the interests of a religious group. No membership is required to relate to spirit. [...] We cannot return to organized religion of dogmatic theology in their old, premodern forms."

CPSIA information can be obtained at www.ICGtesting.com
259965BV00004BA/2/P